Complex Surgical Cases of the LIMBIC SYSTEM

System requirement:

Windows:

- Operating System:
  - Windows Vista or above
  - Macintosh OS X or above
- Recommended Web Browser – Google Chrome & Mozilla Firefox
- Essential plugins – Java & Flash player
  - If facing problems in viewing content – enable/re-install Java plugin on your web browser setting.
  - If Videos don't show up – enable/re-install Flash Player or manage Flash setting on your web browser settings.
  - You can test Java and Flash by using the links from the help section of the CD/DVD.

Accompanying CD/DVD Rom is compatible and playable only in Computers and not in DVD player.

CD/DVD has Autorun function *(only for Windows based systems)*. If Autorun feature doesn't works, then follow the steps below to access the contents manually:

Windows:

- Click on My Computer
- Select the CD/DVD drive and click open/explore – this will show list of files in the CD/DVD
- Find and double click file – "launch.html"

Mac:

Double click the file "launch.html" located on the root after inserting the CD/DVD. The Mac OSX operating system does not support an Autorun feature.

For more information about troubleshoot of Autorun click on: http://support.microsoft.com/kb/330135

Complex Surgical Cases of the LIMBIC SYSTEM

Editors

Sepehr Sani MD
Assistant Professor
Department of Neurosurgery
Rush University Medical Center
Chicago, Illinois, USA

Mustafa K Baskaya MD
Professor
Department of Neurological Surgery
University of Wisconsin-Madison School of Medicine
Madison, Wisconsin, USA

Richard W Byrne MD
Chairman
Department of Neurosurgery
Rush University Medical Center
Chicago, Illinois, USA

Foreword
Aviva Abosch MD PhD

JAYPEE *The Health Sciences Publisher*
New Delhi | London | Panama

Jaypee Brothers Medical Publishers (P) Ltd

Headquarters

Jaypee Brothers Medical Publishers (P) Ltd
4838/24, Ansari Road, Daryaganj
New Delhi 110 002, India
Phone: +91-11-43574357
Fax: +91-11-43574314
E-mail: jaypee@jaypeebrothers.com

Overseas Offices

JP Medical Ltd
83, Victoria Street, London
SW1H 0HW (UK)
Phone: +44 20 3170 8910
Fax: +44 (0)20 3008 6180
E-mail: info@jpmedpub.com

Jaypee-Highlights Medical Publishers Inc
City of Knowledge, Bld. 235, 2nd Floor, Clayton
Panama City, Panama
Phone: +1 507-301-0496
Fax: +1 507-301-0499
E-mail: cservice@jphmedical.com

Jaypee Brothers Medical Publishers (P) Ltd
17/1-B, Babar Road, Block-B, Shaymali
Mohammadpur, Dhaka-1207
Bangladesh
Mobile: +08801912003485
E-mail: jaypeedhaka@gmail.com

Jaypee Brothers Medical Publishers (P) Ltd
Bhotahity, Kathmandu, Nepal
Phone +977-9741283608
E-mail: kathmandu@jaypeebrothers.com

Website: www.jaypeebrothers.com
Website: www.jaypeedigital.com

Inquiries for bulk sales may be solicited at: jaypee@jaypeebrothers.com

Complex Surgical Cases of the Limbic System

First Edition: **2017**

ISBN 978-93-86261-44-1

Printed at Sanat Printers

Dedication

We would like to dedicate this book to our patients and their families.

Contributors

Emel Avci MD
Visiting Research Professor
Department of Neurological Surgery
University of Wisconsin-Madison School of Medicine
Madison, Wisconsin, USA

Ilhan Aydin MD
Research Fellow
Department of Neurological Surgery
University of Wisconsin-Madison School of Medicine
Madison, Wisconsin, USA

Mustafa K Baskaya MD
Professor
Department of Neurological Surgery
University of Wisconsin-Madison School of Medicine
Madison, Wisconsin, USA

Richard W Byrne MD
Chairman
Department of Neurosurgery
Rush University Medical Center
Chicago, Illinois, USA

Ulas Cikla MD
Research Fellow
Department of Neurological Surgery
University of Wisconsin-Madison School of Medicine
Madison, Wisconsin, USA

Demi Dawkins MD
Resident
Department of Neurological Surgery
University of Wisconsin-Madison School of Medicine
Madison, Wisconsin, USA

Carter S Gerard MD
Resident
Department of Neurosurgery
Rush University Medical Center
Chicago, Illinois, USA

Sahin Hanalioglu MD
Research Fellow
Department of Neurological Surgery
University of Wisconsin-Madison School of Medicine
Madison, Wisconsin, USA

Hakan Ozalp MD
Research Fellow
Department of Neurological Surgery
University of Wisconsin-Madison School of Medicine
Madison, Wisconsin, USA

Vikas K Parmar MD
Resident
Department of Neurological Surgery
University of Wisconsin-Madison School of Medicine
Madison, Wisconsin, USA

Sepehr Sani MD
Assistant Professor
Department of Neurosurgery
Rush University Medical Center
Chicago, Illinois, USA

Kyle Swanson MD
Clinical Fellow
Department of Neurological Surgery
University of Wisconsin-Madison School of Medicine
Madison, Wisconsin, USA

Joshua T Wewel MD
Resident
Department of Neurosurgery
Rush University Medical Center
Chicago, Illinois, USA

Foreword

The past decade has witnessed an unprecedented interest in limbic system diseases and their treatments, as functional imaging and neuromodulation of limbic circuitry have gained sway diagnostically and therapeutically, and improvements in operative technique have made approaches to this region increasingly more feasible. Epilepsy, tumor, vascular, and stereotactic neurosurgeons need to understand thoroughly the complex regional anatomy and relationships of the limbic system with the brainstem, diencephalon, and associated vasculature, in order to navigate safely in this region. Unfortunately, and owing to the inherent complexity of this region, it is difficult to find a single compendium of practical surgical knowledge about the limbic system.

Drs Sani, Baskaya, and Byrne have admirably filled this currently unmet need by delivering a comprehensive and beautifully illustrated text that supplies the reader with practical, surgically based, step-by-step descriptions of complex cases in the limbic and paralimbic systems—including temporal, insular and cingulate regions. They begin this journey with a careful review of the embryological development and anatomy of the limbic system, and then methodically tackle the relevant surgical approaches and indications. Using a combination of cadaveric specimens, imaging, and intraoperative photos, to illustrate their clinical experience, the authors provide an unparalleled guide for the field. The information provided in Surgery of the Limbic System serves as a crucial pre-operative guide to surgeons seeking more in-depth information about these regions, whether for epilepsy, tumor, vascular, or stereotactic neurosurgery.

Aviva Abosch MD PhD
Vice Chair for Research
Department of Neurosurgery
Professor of Neurosurgery and Neurology
Director
Department of Stereotactic and Epilepsy Surgery
University of Colorado School of Medicine
Aurora, Colorado, USA
Past-President
American Society for Stereotactic and Functional Neurosurgery

Preface

The limbic and paralimbic areas of the human brain hold profound fascination for both neuroscientists and neurosurgeons. The essential functions of the connections necessitate maintaining functions of the limbic and paralimbic structures, an important goal of surgery in this region. These critically important neuropsychological functional connections are often compromised by the pathology of the mesial temporal lobe, thus making surgery in this region safe, as the deficit created by the pathology is typically not worsened by surgery. The fact that much of the regional pathology is benign, but the conditions they cause, such as epilepsy are not, makes operating in this area a common challenge for neurosurgeons. The unique, obscure, and buried anatomy, the critical surrounding neurovascular structures of limbic and paralimbic archi- and paleo-cortex and the varied, complex pathology makes surgery of this region challenging in the best of circumstances for the most experienced surgeons. For these many reasons, we have dedicated a large portion of our practices, career and research to the mastery of surgery in this region.

The goal in producing this textbook is to pass on to practitioners—neurosurgeons, neurologists, neuroradiologists and neuroscientists—a comprehensive text to act as a compass when confronting limbic and paralimbic pathology. Because limbic pathology is not on the surface, the textbook describes the complex regional anatomy in a practical way for surgeons who must rely on local landmarks more than image guidance. The essential anatomical fiducials available in the limbic lobe are described in great detail, as they are the key to safe surgery in this region. In addition, because the limbic lobe is not visible on the surface of the brain, the issue of choosing the safest surgical approach is paramount. Much attention to surgical approach is included in this text. Finally, the diversity of pathology that is found in this region is addressed. From mesial temporal sclerosis, to glioma, to vascular lesions, all common pathologies are covered.

Richard W Byrne MD

Acknowledgments

The production of this book owes significant gratitude to the many who have shaped out interest and knowledge in the field of neurosurgery. We would like to thank Dr Andre Olivier who sparked the interest in limbic neurosurgery. Drs Walter Whisler and the late Roy AE Bakay who provided tremendous mentorship and serves as role models for excellence. The physical production of this work would not have been possible without the dedicated efforts of Anthony Serici at Rush University's department of Anatomy and Cell Biology.

Lastly, we would like to thank Mr Jitendar P Vij (Group Chairman), Mr Ankit Vij (Group President), Ms Chetna Malhotra Vohra (Associate Director—Content Strategy), Nikita Chauhan (Development Editor) and the entire team of Jaypee Brothers Medical Publishers, New Delhi, India for their tireless efforts in producing the book in its final form.

Contents

Introduction

The limbic and paralimbic areas of the human brain hold profound fascination for both neuroscientists and neurosurgeons. Maintaining the essential neuropsychological functions of the limbic and paralimbic structures is an important goal of surgery in this region. These critically important neuropsychological functional connections are often compromised by the pathology of the mesial temporal lobe, thus making surgery in this region safe, as the deficit created by the pathology is typically not worsened by surgery. The fact that much of the regional pathology is benign, but the conditions they cause, such as epilepsy are not, makes operating in this area a common challenge for neurosurgeons. The unique, obscure, and buried anatomy, the critical surrounding neurovascular structures of limbic and paralimbic archi- and paleo-cortex and the varied, complex pathology makes surgery of this region challenging in the best of circumstances for the most experienced surgeons. For these many reasons, we have dedicated a large portion of our practices, career and research to the mastery of surgery in this region.

The goal in producing this textbook is to pass on to practitioners-neurosurgeons, neurologists, neuroradiologists and neuroscientists a comprehensive text to act as a compass when confronting limbic and paralimbic pathology. Because limbic pathology is not on the surface, the textbook describes the complex regional anatomy in a practical way for surgeons who must rely on local landmarks more than image guidance. The essential anatomical fiducials available in the limbic lobe are described in great detail, as they are the key to safe surgery in this region. In addition, because the limbic lobe is not visible on the surface of the brain, the issue of choosing the safest surgical approach is paramount. Much attention to surgical approach is included in this text. Finally, the diversity of pathology that is found in this region is addressed. From mesial temporal sclerosis, to glioma, to vascular lesions, all common pathologies are covered.

CHAPTER 1

Embryology

Sepehr Sani, Joshua T Wewel, Richard W Byrne

INTRODUCTION

One of the most dramatic developmental changes of the central nervous system is that seen in the limbic system. Various structures of the adult limbic system encompass every lobe as well as the brainstem with interconnections via fiber tracks that at times travel almost circumferential distances. The embryologic development of the human limbic system is evolutionarily old and has remained remarkably consistent over time and across most mammalian species. The formation of various structures of the limbic system in conjunction with the surrounding brain development helps explain the form and function of the adult limbic system. A thorough understanding of the limbic embryologic development is critical to the neurosurgeon's ability to operate safely within its structures.

STRUCTURE AND DEVELOPMENT OF LIMBIC SYSTEM

The limbic system extends from the medial surface of the frontal lobe to the temporal lobe, comprising a series of four C-shaped structures that are separated by sulci or remnants (Fig. 1.1). The outermost "C" arch is formed sequentially by the subcallosal area, cingulate gyrus, parahippocampal gyrus, and uncus. The inner arch is formed by the paraterminal gyrus, indusium griseum, tail of hippocampus, dentate gyrus, and Ammon's horn.[1-4] A long sulcus between these two arches, the callosal sulcus and the hippocampal fissure, defines the third arch. The fourth and final arch is formed by the fimbria and fornix.[2,4,5] The anatomic complexity of the limbic structures is reflected by their embryological development and an overview is presented in the following text.

Developmentally, the limbic system arises from the telencephalon and diencephalon.[4-6] Examination of the gray matter architecture reveals that most structures have a three layered cortex. The dentate gyrus and Ammon's horn have a trilaminar type of cortex which gradually transitions to a neocortical six layer cortex in the entorhinal area of the parahippocampal gyrus.[4,7]

Hippocampus

The hippocampus first appears at the dorsomedial wall of the cerebral hemisphere adjacent to the lamina terminalis at around day 37 of gestation[4-6,8,9] and is the first cortical area to differentiate.[8-10] This structure forms a continuous bulge into the inferomedial wall of the lateral

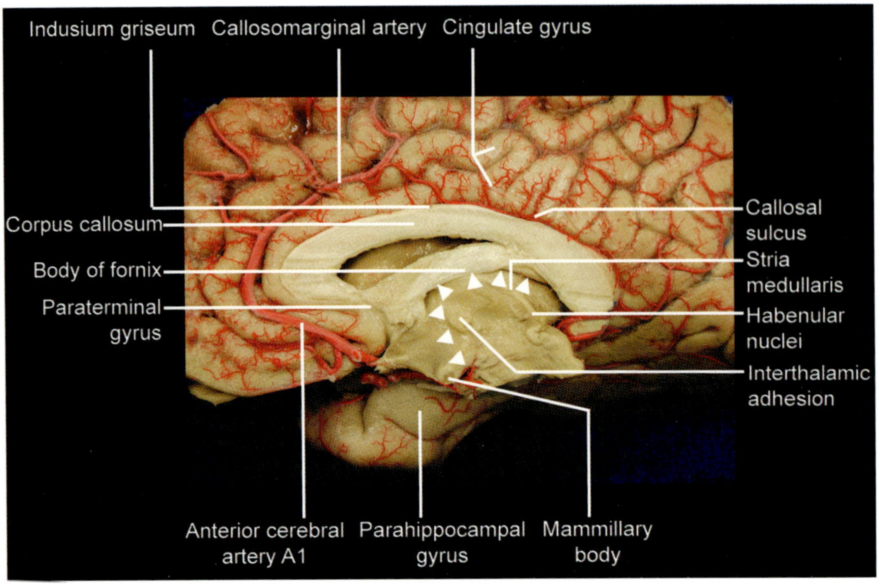

Fig. 1.1: Mesial surface of brain demonstrating the adult pathway of the four limbic arches. The outermost arch is formed by the cingulate gyrus, which merges with and becomes the parahippocampal gyrus. The inner arch is formed by the indusium griseum, which is the adult remnant of the hippocampus. This structure is continuous with the tail of hippocampus, dentate gyrus, and Ammon's horn. The callosal sulcus, which becomes the hippocampal fissure, defines the third arch. The fourth and final arch is formed by the fimbria and fornix (white arrowheads).

ventricle as it extends in crescent fashion into the temporal tip where the temporal lobe forms. At week 10 of gestation, the hippocampus forms a large part of the cerebral hemisphere.[11]

As the corpus callosum begins to develop around 14 weeks' gestation, the anterior hippocampus regresses and the temporal portion remains as the most developed part.[8,11] By 17 weeks, the paraterminal gyrus and indusium griseum are the only remnants of the anterior hippocampus. In the temporal lobe, the anterior tip of the hippocampus is separated from the developing amygdala by the uncal recess of the temporal horn. The body of the hippocampus forms the inferomedial border of the temporal horn with its subependymal superior surface covered by the alveus (Figs. 1.2A to D). The hippocampal tail extends around the splenium of the corpus callosum and forms the indusium griseum.[3,12,13] The indusium griseum and its associated white matter bundles (medial and lateral longitudinal striae) are intimately applied to the surface of the corpus callosum.[4,14] Anteriorly, the indusium griseum extends around the genu of the corpus callosum to merge with the paraterminal gyrus.[3,4,13,15]

The hippocampal fissure is first seen at about 55 days' gestation but is not well formed until 10 weeks.[8,16] It forms as a result of the differential growth of Ammon's horn compared to the dentate gyrus.[10,11,16] By 15 weeks (Figs. 1.2A to D), the most developed part of the fissure is in the temporal lobe.[8,11] With continued growth of the dentate gyrus, the hippocampal fissure deepens and eventually fuses together. A remnant cavity of this can be seen in 10% of the normal population in MRI studies.[7,17] The medial hemispheric part of the fissure eventually becomes the callosal sulcus separating the indusium griseum from the cingulate gyrus.[2,5] In the temporal lobe, the hippocampal fissure runs parallel to the choroidal fissure[5] and merges into the uncal sulcus.[17]

Parahippocampal Gyrus

The parahippocampal gyrus forms the inferomedial surface of the temporal lobe in the adult form. Developmentally, the hippocampal fissure forms the superior border of the parahippocampal gyrus. On the lateral side, the collateral sulcus separates it from the occipitotemporal gyrus. Beginning at 13 weeks and soon after, the parahippocampal gyrus undergoes rapid growth and expansion, essentially causing it to rotate in the inferomedial direction, covering the hippocampus and hippocampal fissure.

Fornix and Mammillary Body

The fornix is the main efferent fiber tract from the hippocampus. The majority of fibers arise from the subiculum and Ammon's horn,[13,18] travel over the subependymal ventricular surface as the alveus and merge as the fimbria. The fimbria lies superior to the dentate gyrus and is

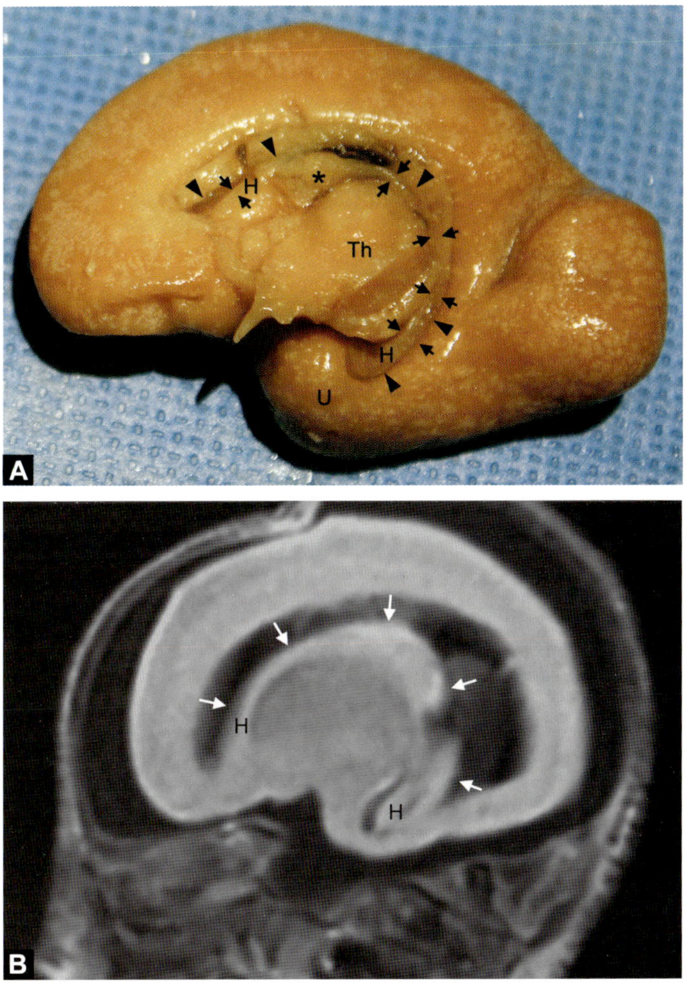

Figs. 1.2A and B

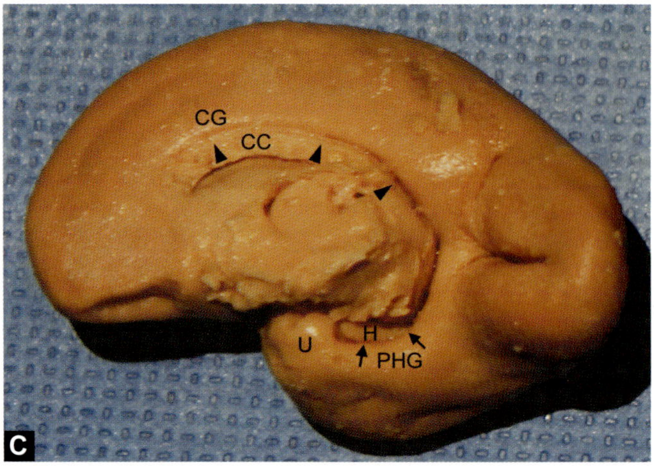

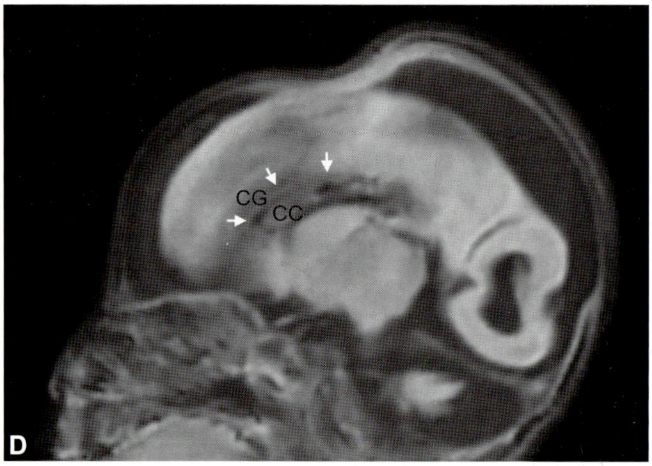

Figs. 1.2A to D: Photographs and MRI images of the medial surface of the embryological cerebral hemispheres. (A) The medial surface of an approximately 14-week-old embryo. The hippocampus (*H*) extends from the temporal lobe to the frontal lobe (small arrows). The prominent hippocampal sulcus is readily visible (large arrowheads). The uncus (*U*) has an anterior position but has not fully turned to cover the hippocampus medially. (*Th*: Thalamus;*: Area affected by dissection) (B) Reformatted sagittal oblique MRI image of the same specimen demonstrating the hippocampus (*H*) and the hippocampal sulcus (small arrows). (C) The medial surface of an approximately 17-week-old specimen. The corpus callosum (*CC*) is partially formed and the hippocampal remnant along the sulcus of the corpus callosum (arrowheads) is visible along the frontoparietal region. The cingulate gyrus (*CG*) is now visible. The hippocampal sulcus (small arrows) is less visible as the uncus (*U*) assumes a more medial position. Early formation of the parahippocampal gyrus (*PHG*) is also seen at this time. (D) Sagittal MRI image of the same specimen. The hippocampal remnant is seen (arrows) along the forming sulcus of the corpus callosum.

separated from it by the fimbriodentate fissure. Posteriorly, the fimbria increases in thickness, becoming the crura of fornix. Anteriorly, the crura form a triangular sheet of fibers called the commissure of the fornix. The crura then join to from the body of the fornix, which continue on to becoming the columns of the fornix before dividing proximal to the anterior commissure to the precommissural and postcommissural fibers. The precommissural fibers terminate in the septal area, diagonal band of Broca, lateral preoptic area, and anterior hypothalamus. The postcommissural fibers terminate in the mammillary bodies.

The fibers of the fornix appear at 8 weeks' gestation. The commissure of the fornix begins to appear around 10 weeks and by 13.5 weeks, the alveus is visible in the subependymal surface, and the fimbriodentate fissure is present.[8] The fornix and hippocampus can be seen as separate entities after 16 weeks gestational age.[14] The mammillary bodies, which are diencephalic in origin, arise as a single rounded protuberance from the floor of the hypothalamus. Around the 3rd month of gestation, the mammillary bodies are divided by a median furrow, forming the left and right sides.[4-6]

Septal Area

The septal area is an important part of the limbic system and serves as an area of interconnection for various anatomic nuclei. The area includes the subcallosal gyrus, paraterminal gyrus, septal nuclei, olfactory stria, and the diagonal band of broca.[5,13,15] This region is located on the medial surface of the frontal lobe, inferior to the corpus callosum and anterior to the lamina terminalis.[4,15]

The septal area is a telencephalic structure that first appears at 37 days' gestational age.[8] The septal nuclei and some of the fiber connections can be identified at about 47 days' gestation. By the 3rd month of gestation, the septal nuclei are well-developed and lie below the corpus callosum and anterior to the septum pellucidum near their adult anatomic position.[8]

Amygdala

The amygdala is an almond-shaped collection of nuclei that have both olfactory and limbic functions.[19] Although in the adult brain, the uncus which encompasses the amygdala and the hippocampus has an intimate anatomic relationship, as will be explained here, the two structures are distinct and develop separately during gestation. The amygdala arises from the corpus striatum embryologically and remains directly connected to the putamen superiorly and the tail of the caudate nucleus that ends in the amygdala.[4,5,13,18] The amygdala is divided into two major masses of nuclei: (1) the corticomedial and (2) basolateral nuclear group.

Developmentally, the amygdala is the first part of the corpus striatum to appear as a thickening next to the primitive hippocampal formation at about 35 days' gestation. As it develops, the amygdala migrates from being directly posterior to the lateral ventricle to its ventral and anterior temporal location; and it rotates medially such that nuclei that were originally lateral become basal and ventral in position.[8,20,21] This parallels the development of the temporal horn and medial rotation of the temporal pole. This development continues until the adult uncus assumes its anteromedial temporal position.

Insula

The sylvian fold and insular region begin to develop by gestation week 18. This is followed by the development of the central insular sulcus, which is visible on the surface before the

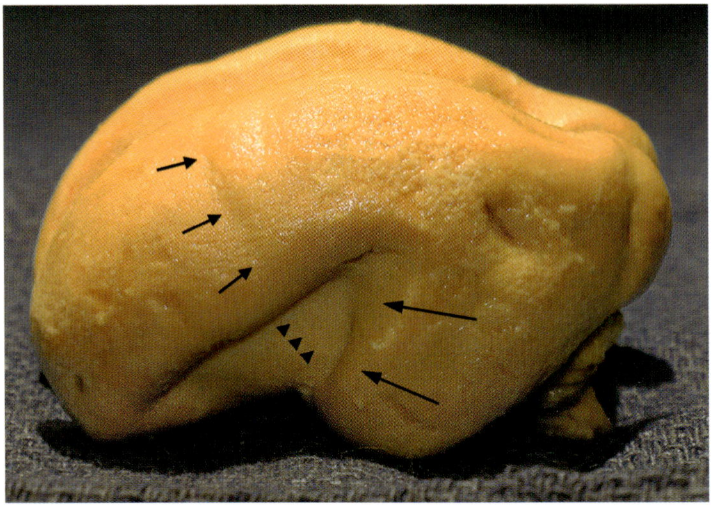

Fig. 1.3: Lateral surface of the embryological hemisphere at 19-week gestation age. The frontoparietal central sulcus (small arrows) is visible and is aligned with the developing central insular sulcus (arrowheads). As the temporal lobe continues to fold and join the frontotemporal opercula (large arrows), the insula assumes its adult hidden position.

temporal and frontal lobes fold. The central insular sulcus corresponds to the location and development of the central sulcus of the frontoparietal lobes (Fig. 1.3). As development continues by 22 weeks' gestation, the insula becomes narrower and less visible due to the posterior-to-anterior folding of the temporal lobe against the parietal and frontal opercula. The Sylvian fissure becomes anatomically visible and completely closed by 27 weeks gestation, at which point the insula is no longer visible.

CONCLUSION

The developmental anatomy of the limbic system is complex. A detailed understanding of the sequential development of various structures allows for an understanding of the adult structures including the four C-shaped arches, lying in an oblique sagittal plane and extending from the temporal pole to the medial surface of the frontal lobe.

REFERENCES

1. Duvernoy H. The Human Brain: Surface, Three Dimensional Sectional Anatomy and MRI. New York: Springer-Verlag; 1991.
2. Mark LP, Daniels DL, Naidich TP, Borne JA. Limbic system anatomy: an overview. Am J Neuroradiol. 1993;14(2):349-52.
3. Naidich TP, Daniels DL, Haughton VM, Pech P, Williams A, Pojunas K, et al. Hippocampal formation and related structures of the limbic lobe: anatomic-MR correlation. Part II. Sagittal sections. Radiology. 1987;162(3):755-61.
4. Gray FRS, Wolff K, Winkelman R. Gray's Anatomy. Philadelphia: WB Saunders; 1980.
5. Carpenter MB. Human Neuroanatomy, 8th edition. Baltimore: Williams & Wilkins; 1983.

6. O'Rahilly RR, F Müller. Human Embryology and Teratology. New York: Wiley-Liss; 1992.
7. Bronen RA, Cheung G. MRI of the normal hippocampus. Magn Reson Imaging. 1991;9(4):497-500.
8. Lemire RJ, Loeser JD, Leech RW, et al. Normal and Abnormal Development of the Human Nervous System. Hagerstown, MD: Harper & Row; 1975.
9. O'Rahilly MF. The Embryonic Human Brain: An Atlas of Developmental Stages. New York: Wiley-Liss; 1994.
10. Humphrey T. The development of the human hippocampal formation correlated with some aspects of its phylogenetic history. In: Evolution of the Forebrain: Phylogenesis and Ontogenesis of the Forebrain. New York: Plenum Press; 1967.
11. Kier EL, Fulbright RK, Bronen RA. Limbic lobe embryology and anatomy: dissection and MR of the medial surface of the fetal cerebral hemisphere. Am J Neuroradiol. 1995;16(9):1847-53.
12. Mark LP, Daniels DL, Naidich TP, et al, Borne JA. The hippocampus. Am J Neuroradiol. 1993;14(3):709-12.
13. Naidich TP, Daniels DL, Haughton VM, Williams A, Pojunas K, Palacios E. Hippocampal formation and related structures of the limbic lobe: anatomic-MR correlation. Part I. Surface features and coronal sections. Radiology. 1987;162(3):747-54.
14. Sitoh YY, Tien RD. The limbic system. An overview of the anatomy and its development. Neuroimaging Clin N Am. 1997;7(1):1-10.
15. Mark LP, Daniels DL, Naidich TP, et al, Maas E. Anatomic moment. The septal area. Am J Neuroradiol. 1994;15(2):273-6.
16. Humphrey T. The development of the human hippocampal fissure. J Anat. 1967;101(Pt 4):655-76.
17. Hayman LA, Hinck VC. Adult cerebrum. In: Clinical Brain Imaging: Normal Structure and Functional Anatomy. St. Louis: Mosby-Year Book; 1992.
18. Nieuwenhuys R, Voogd J, Van Huijzen C. The Human Central Nervous System: A Synopsis and Atlas, 3rd edition. New York: Springer-Verlag; 1988.
19. Kretschmann H-J, W Weinrich. Cranial Neuroimaging and Clinical Neuroanatomy, 2nd edition. New York: Thieme; 1992.
20. Humphrey T. The development of the human amygdala during early embryonic life. J Comp Neurol. 1968;132(1):135-65.
21. Humphrey T. The development of the human amygdaloid complex. The Neurobiology of the Amygdala. New York: Plenum Press; 1972.

CHAPTER 2

Anatomy

Sepehr Sani

INTRODUCTION

The limbic system is derived from cortical and subcortical structures surrounding the thalamus and basal ganglia arched in a "C"-shaped orientation. This is a reflection of the structures' embryological development as described in the previous chapter.

The neocortical limbic structures include the temporal gyri, parahippocampal gyrus, subiculum and uncus, cingulate gyrus, and the insular gyri. The paleocortical and subcortical structures that are part of the limbic circuit and communicate with the cortical areas are the hippocampus (including the dentate gyrus), fornix and fimbria, amygdala, habenula, mammillary body, septal nuclei, and portions of the thalamus, hypothalamus, and midbrain (Fig. 2.1).

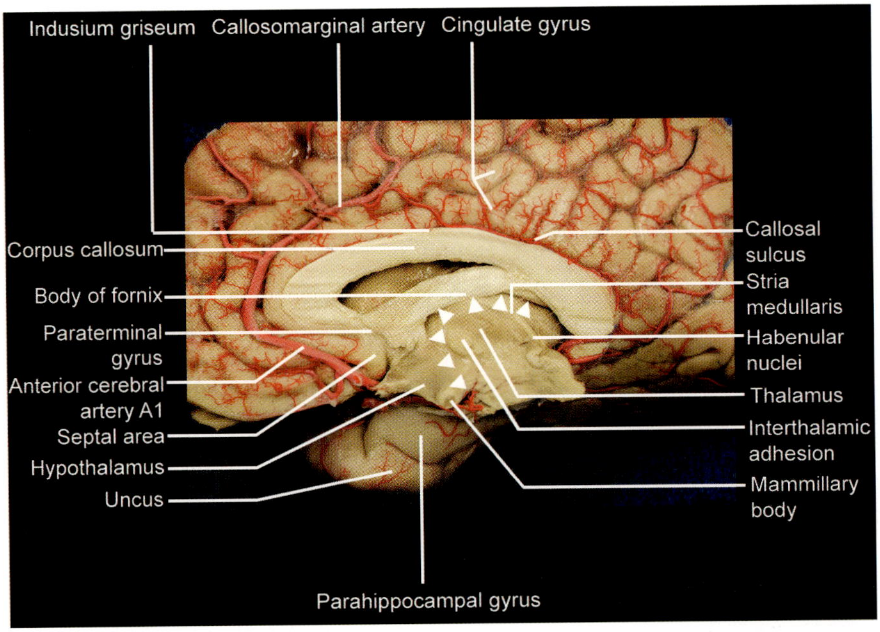

Fig. 2.1: Mesial surface of brain demonstrating the key components of the limbic system.

The unique anatomical location of the limbic structures, their inter-relationship, and the intimate association with the deep arterial and venous anatomy render them particularly challenging in the operative environment. This chapter will detail the surgical anatomy of each structure along with the pertinent vascular anatomy as it applies to the neurosurgeon.

TEMPORAL LOBE

The temporal lobe is unique due to its histology, anatomy and close relationship with commonly used surgical corridors.

Histology

Histologically, the temporal lobe is characterized by a transition from the three layered cortex of the hippocampus and amygdala to the six layered mesocortex of the parahippocampal gyrus in the basal temporal lobe, to the six layered neocortex including the superior, middle, interior, and transverse temporal gyri and the fusiform gyrus.

Anatomy

The temporal lobe is separated from the frontal and parietal lobes by the sylvian fissure. Posteriorly, the temporal lobe continues with the occipital lobe at the lingual gyrus. The temporal lobe is connected superiorly to the insula through the temporal stem, anteromedially to the basal ganglia via the amygdala and anterolaterally to the basal forebrain structures via the limen insula. The choroidal fissure divides the medial portion of temporal lobe behind the uncus from the thalamus.

The temporal lobe consists of four surfaces: (1) the lateral surface, (2) the basal surface, (3) the superior surface, and (4) the mesial surface. The lateral surface is composed of the superior, middle, and inferior temporal gyri, separated by the superior and inferior temporal sulci (Fig. 2.2). The basal surface (Fig. 2.3) is represented lateral to medial by the occipitotemporal sulcus which separates the inferior temporal gyrus from the fusiform gyrus, the collateral sulcus, and the parahippocampal gyrus. The superior surface (Fig. 2.4) consists of the planum polare, Heschl's gyrus, and the planum temporale from anterior to posterior.

Superior Surface

The superior surface of the temporal lobe, also referred to as the temporal operculum, constitutes the inferior wall of the sylvian fissure. From anterior to posterior, it is composed of planum polare, Heschl's gyrus, and planum temporale.

The planum polare is a depression on the anterior surface of the superior temporal lobe. It is bordered by the uncus anteromedially and Heschl's gyrus posteriorly. Heschl's gyrus has a distinct medial to lateral direction and is bordered by the planum polare anteriorly and planum temporale posteriorly. Laterally, it fuses with the superior temporal gyrus. The junction between Heschl's gyrus and the superior temporal gyrus usually occurs at the level of the acoustic meatus on the coronal plane and is not visible on the surface anatomy of the brain.

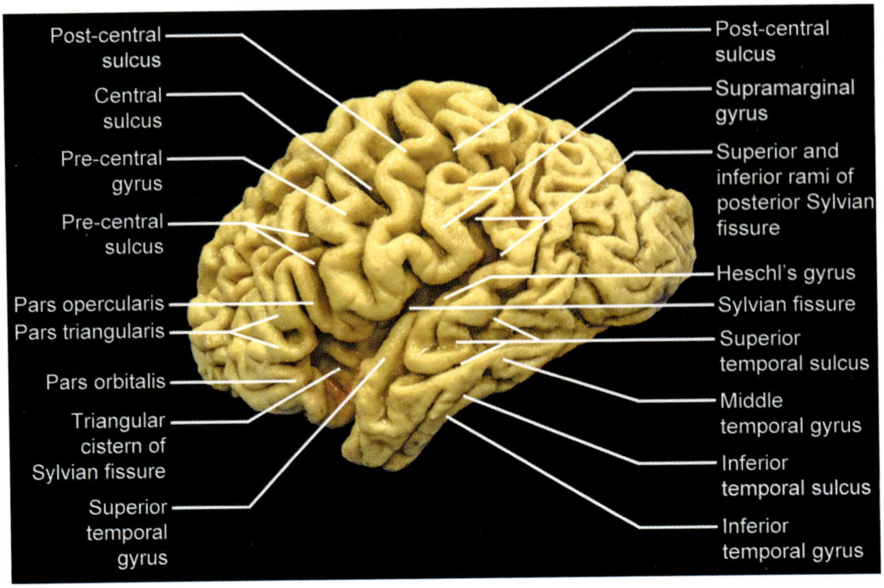

Fig. 2.2: Lateral surface of the left hemisphere demonstrating the surface anatomy of the temporal lobe. The sylvian fissure divides the temporal lobe from the frontal and parietal opercula. Note the opening in the fissure allowing visualization of Heschl's gyrus, which joins the superior temporal gyrus on the lateral surface of temporal lobe. The posterior extension of the sylvian fissure ends in the superior and inferior rami, which are, in turn, surrounded by the supramarginal gyrus. The superior and middle temporal gyri are divided by the superior temporal sulcus. The middle and inferior temporal gyri, in turn, are divided by the inferior temporal sulcus.

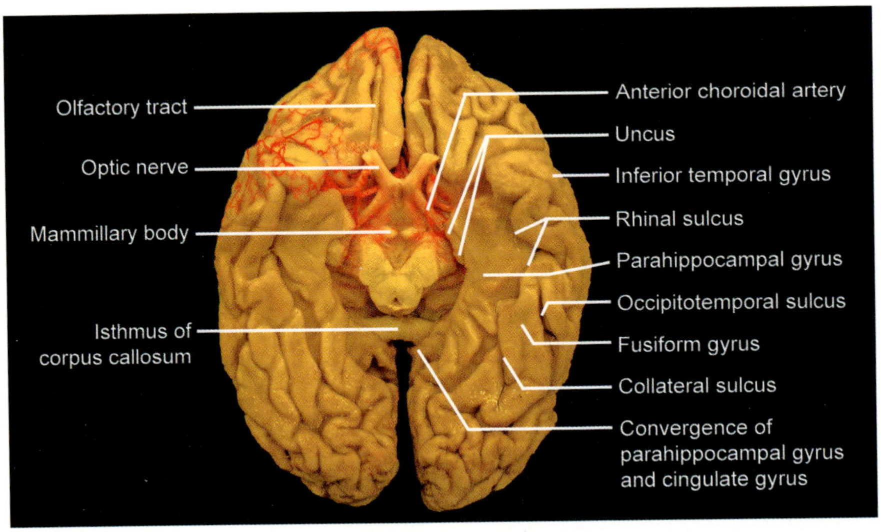

Fig. 2.3: Basal view of the brain with the relevant temporal lobe anatomy labeled. In sequence from lateral to medial, the inferior temporal gyrus is separated from the fusiform gyrus by the occipitotemporal sulcus, which, in turn, is separated from the parahippocampal gyrus by the very deep and consistent collateral sulcus.

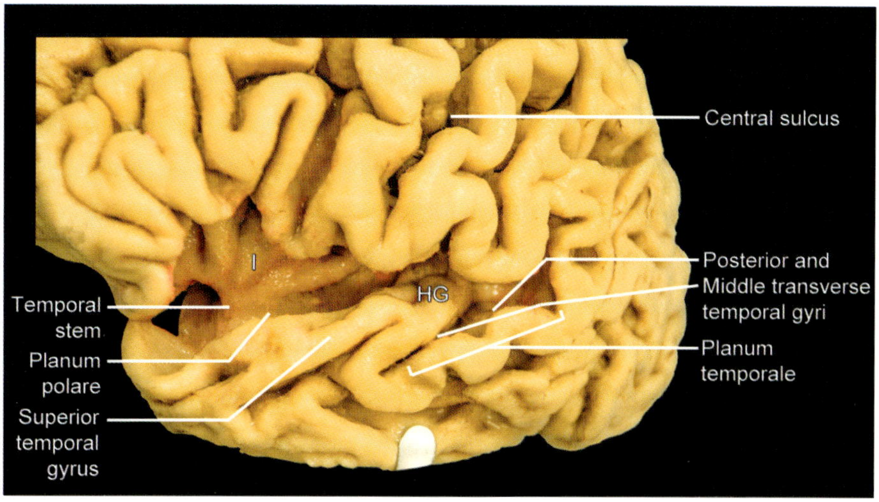

Fig. 2.4: View of the superior temporal lobe of the left hemisphere. The Sylvian fissure has been opened. Anteriorly, the planum polare is seen as a depression on the anterior surface of the superior temporal lobe. Note the insula (I) in background and temporal stem. Heschl's gyrus (HG) is a distinct transverse gyrus that connects with the superior temporal gyrus and divides the superior surface of the temporal lobe from the planum polare anteriorly and planum temporal posteriorly. The planum temporale consists of the anterior (Heschl's), middle and posterior transverse temporal gyri.

However, Heschl's gyrus is characteristically identified radiographically by its characteristic "hump" (Fig. 2.5).

Mesial Surface

The parahippocampal gyrus runs anterior to posterior along the basomedial aspect of the temporal lobe (Fig. 2.6). It bends at its anterior end in the posteromedial direction to form the uncus. Posteriorly, the parahippocampal gyrus is divided by the calcarine fissure from the isthmus of the cingulate gyrus. Medially, the parahippocampal gyrus (the subiculum component) wraps around the tentorial edge. On the superior side, the parahippocampal gyrus is separated from the dentate gyrus by the hippocampal sulcus. Laterally, it is limited by the collateral sulcus; an important surgical landmark since it abuts the lateral edge of the temporal horn (Fig. 2.7). The anterior portion of the parahippocampal gyrus is the entorhinal area which is bordered laterally by the rhinal sulcus.

Uncus

The name 'uncus' means 'hook' and is derived from the curving of the parahippocampal gyrus in the posteromedial direction. There is a sulcus between the parahippocampal gyrus and uncus proper, the uncal notch. On the superior side, the amygdalar portion of the uncus is continuous with the globus pallidus. Laterally, the uncus is separated from the temporal pole by the rhinal sulcus. The medial edge of the uncus is free and abuts the carotid cistern anteriorly and the tentorium posteriorly.

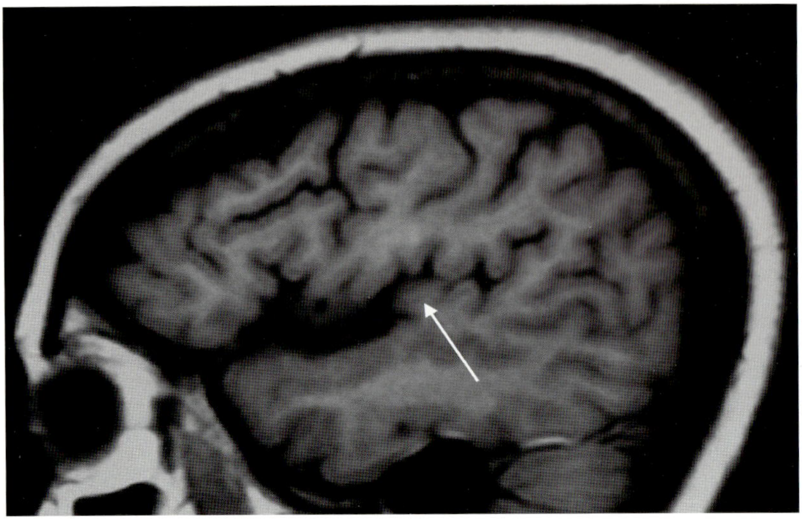

Fig. 2.5: Magnetic resonance imaging (MRI) of brain. Sagittal T1-weighted image demonstrating the characteristic location and "hump" of Heschl's gyrus (arrow).

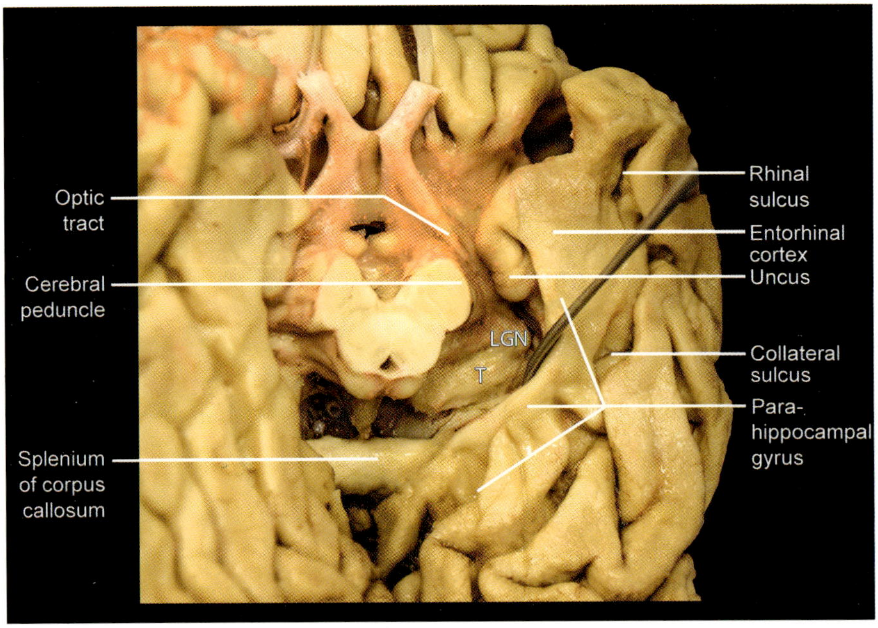

Fig. 2.6: Basal oblique visualization of the left hemisphere. The medial temporal lobe and its surrounding relationships are demonstrated. The anterior portion of the hippocampus forms the entorhinal cortex, which is separated laterally by the rhinal sulcus. The parahippocampal gyrus, bordered laterally by the collateral sulcus, travels along the mesial border of the temporal lobe. Anteriorly, it is encompassed by the uncus. Further posterior, the parahippocampal gyrus is retracted to note the intimate relationship of the lateral geniculate nucleus (LGN) of the thalamus (T) with the mesial portion of the parahippocampal gyrus. The LGN extends dorsolaterally and forms part of the roof to the temporal horn. The parahippocampal gyrus "wraps" around the splenium of the corpus callosum as the cingulate gyrus.

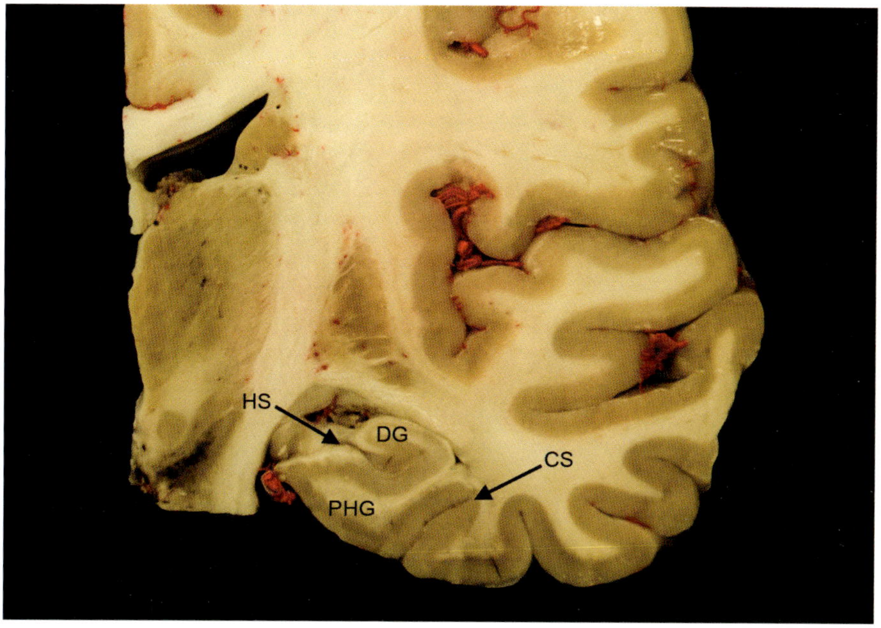

Fig. 2.7: Coronal image of the left hemisphere showing the mesial temporal lobe relationships. The parahippocampal gyrus (PHG) surrounds the mesial side the temporal lobe and is separated from the dentate gyrus (DG) segment of the hippocampus by the hippocampal sulcus (HS). The collateral sulcus (CS) marks the lateral margin of the PHG and its superior border is a very consistent landmark for finding the temporal horn during surgery.

The uncus is composed of five small gyri that, when viewed from the medial surface, resemble the bulges of a pumpkin attached superiorly. From anterior to posterior, the gyri are the semilunar (comprising the amygdala) and ambient, followed by the uncinate gyrus, the band of Giacomini, and the inftralimbic gyrus (Fig. 2.8). The boundary between the semilunar gyrus and the globus pallidus is nondiscrete. Limen insulae is directly anterolateral to this junction. The infralimbic gyrus is of surgical significance as it marks the most posterior gyrus of the uncus. Immediately posterior to this is the choroidal point, where the choroid plexus of the temporal horn begins, and also where the choroidal artery enters the temporal horn through the choroidal fissure (Fig. 2.9). The hippocampal formation is directly posterior to the choroidal point.

Amygdala

The amygdala is composed entirely within the uncus and has an intimate relationship with the anterior wall of the temporal horn (Fig. 2.10). Superiorly, the amygdala blends in with the globus pallidus and is difficult to distinguish surgically. Inferiorly and posteriorly, it forms the anterior wall and the anterior portion of the roof of the temporal horn. The amygdalar complex is composed of several nuclei which are collectively divided into three nuclear groups—(1) the basolateral, (2) the corticomedial, and (3) the central group.

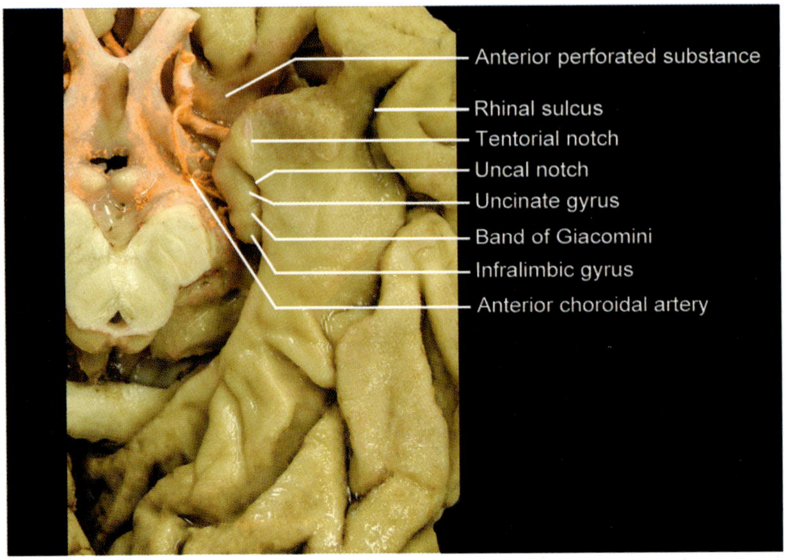

Fig. 2.8: Topographic anatomy of the uncus as viewed from the basal surface of the left hemisphere. The uncus is separated from the anterior hippocampus by a sulcus called the uncal notch. The tentorial notch is also visible and labeled. The uncus proper is composed of five small gyri, three of which are readily visible on this specimen. From anterior to posterior, the uncal gyri are: semilunar (not visualized), ambient (not visualized), uncinated, band of Giacomini, and the infralimbic gyri. The infralimbic gyrus marks the most posterior part of the uncus and is intimately associated with the cerebral peduncle.

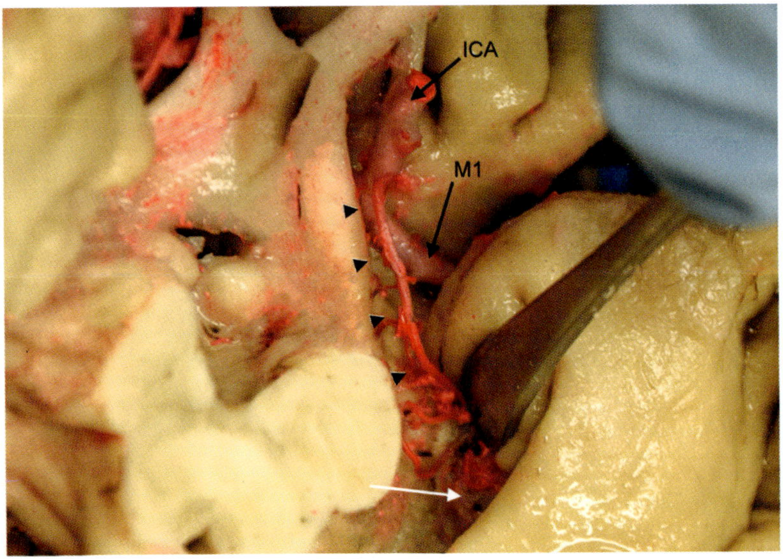

Fig. 2.9: Same specimen as in Figure 2.8 visualized at an oblique angle in order to demonstrate the vascular relationships. The anterior choroidal artery (arrowheads) arises from the internal carotid artery (ICA) before the bifurcation. The M1 segment of the middle cerebral artery is visualized ascending into the Sylvian fissure. The uncus is reflected to reveal the anterior choroidal artery and its tributaries traveling to the choroidal point (white arrow) where they enter the temporal horn to supply the choroid plexus.

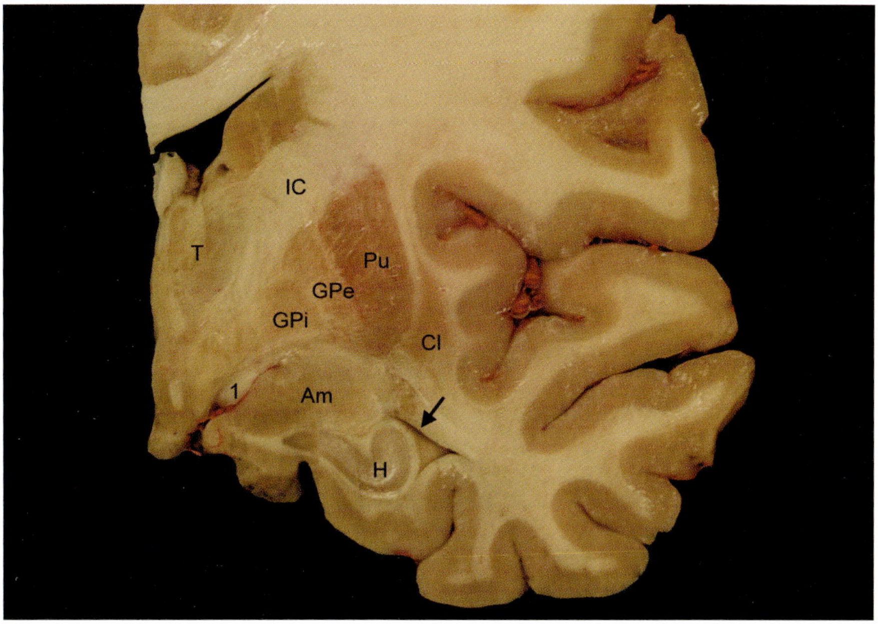

Fig. 2.10: Coronal cross-section of the left hemisphere demonstrating the relationship between the amygdala and the surrounding anatomy, in particular, the basal ganglia. The semilunar gyrus of the uncus contains the amygdala proper (Am). Laterally, the amygdala forms the superomedial roof of the temporal horn (arrow) and is closely associated with the hippocampal head (H). The optic radiation (1) is located between the amygdala laterally and the hypothalamus medially. Superiorly, the amygdala does not have a clear border and is intimately associated with the basal ganglia: the putamen (Pu), globus pallidus pars externa (GPe) and interna (GPi).
(Cl: Claustrum; IC: Internal capsule; T: Thalamus).

Hippocampus

The hippocampus, with its distinct embryological formation from the uncus, occupies the medial and inferior walls of the temporal horn. The hippocampus has three anatomical components: head, body, and tail. The head is the largest part and is located at the medial end of the tip of the temporal horn, characterized by several small digitations (Figs. 2.11 and 2.12). Superiorly, the head abuts the posterior margin of the amygdala which bulges into the temporal horn anteriorly, the head is related to the uncal recess, which is the anterior continuation of the collateral recess. The posterior margin of the hippocampal head and the starting point of the hippocampal body are marked by the formation of choroid plexus, the fimbria, and the choroidal fissure. The body of the hippocampus bends in an anteroposterior direction and gets narrower as it approaches the atrium of the lateral ventricle. Along the course of the hippocampal body, the medial wall of the temporal horn is thin and composed of the choroidal fissure, which is intimately associated with the ambient cistern. As the hippocampal tail approaches the atrium, it gets progressively thinner and fuses with the calcar avis (the bulge on the medial wall of the atrium). The remaining portion of the tail is microscopic and follows the

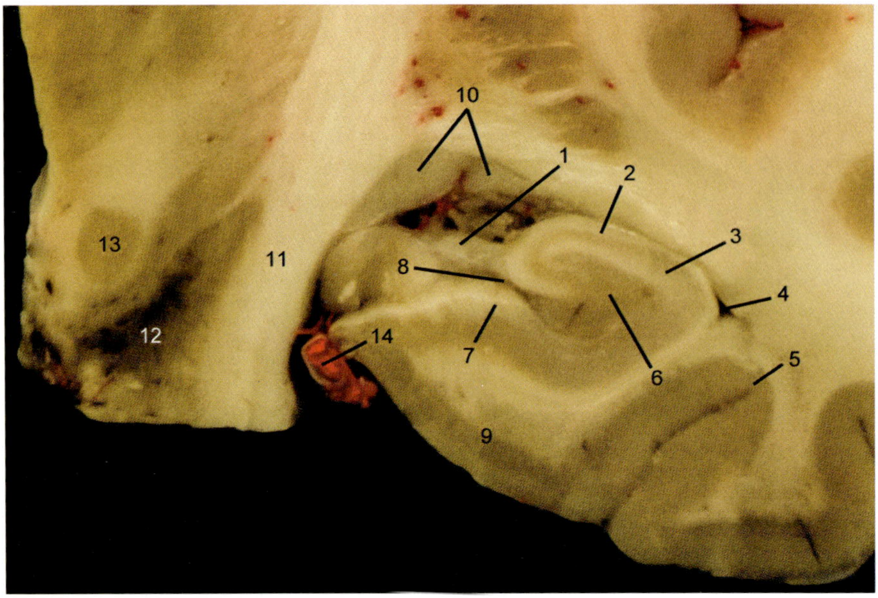

Fig. 2.11: Coronal cross-section of the left hippocampus body. The alveus (2) and Ammon's horn (3) segments of the hippocampus compose the surface visible within the temporal horn (4). Medially, the parahippocampal gyrus (9) merges with the subiculum (7). The parahippocampal gyrus is separated from the hippocampus proper by the hippocampal sulcus (8). 1, fimbria; 2, alveus; 3, Ammon's horn; 4, temporal horn; 5, collateral sulcus; 6, dentate gyrus; 7, subiculum; 8, hippocampal sulcus; 9, parahippocampal gyrus; 10, lateral and medial geniculate nuclei; 11, cerebral peduncle; 12, substantia nigra; 13, red nucleus.

C-shaped pattern around the corpus callosum as the subsplenial gyrus, along with the indusium griseum of the dentate gyrus.

The ventricular surface of the hippocampus is covered by white matter called alveus, which thickens on the medial side of the hippocampus and forms the fimbria of the fornix, another limbic structure that travels in the C-shaped direction around the corpus callosum, carrying the output information of the hippocampus (Fig. 2.11). The fornix wraps around the pulvinar nucleus of thalamus (crus of the fornix), arching anteromedially toward the splenium of the corpus callosum. Anteriorly, the columns of the fornix form the anterior borders of the foramen of Monro. The columns then split rostral to the anterior commissure. The majority of the fibers are postcommissural and are directed around the wall of the third ventricle to reach the mammillary bodies. The precommissural fibers continue onto the basal forebrain structures.

The dentate gyrus encompasses the medial surface of the hippocampus and runs along its course (Fig. 2.11). Inferiorly, the dentate gyrus is separated from the parahippocampal gyrus by the hippocampal sulcus. On its superior side, the fimbrodentate sulcus separates the dentate gyrus from the fimbria of the fornix. The dentate gyrus continues anteriorly with the band of Giacomini of the uncus. Posteriorly, the dentate gyrus follows the C-shaped trajectory of the corpus callosum around the thalamus as the indusium griseum and ends as the paraterminal gyrus.

Temporal Horn and Choroidal Fissure

Because of the anatomical relationships of the temporal horn and choroidal fissure during neurosurgical procedures, such as lateral temporal, trans-sylvian, or occipitotemporal approaches, special mention of relevant anatomy is made here.

Topographically, the temporal horn is located at the level of the middle temporal gyrus anteriorly. As one proceeds posteriorly, the atrium is topographically aligned with the junction of the superior temporal gyrus and the supramarginal gyrus. Perhaps the most important association of the temporal horn is the roof and the optic radiation (Fig. 2.13). Anteriorly, the roof of the temporal horn is part of the temporal stem and as one continues posteriorly, the roof is composed of various traversing fibers including the parietopontine, occipitopontine, occipitocollicular, and occipitotectal fibers. In addition, the acoustic radiation from the medial geniculate body to the superior temporal and Heschl's gyrus and the optic radiation from the lateral geniculate to the occipital lobe form part of the roof of temporal horn. Given the relationship of the fibers running along the roof of the temporal horn with the geniculate nuclei of the thalamus, it is reasonable to consider the thalamus as part of the roof of temporal horn; an important consideration when attempting to enter the temporal horn superiorly such as via a trans-Sylvian approach.

Another important landmark in the temporal horn is the choroidal fissure (Fig. 2.12). It is easily identified during dissection in the temporal horn and can readily orient the neurosur-

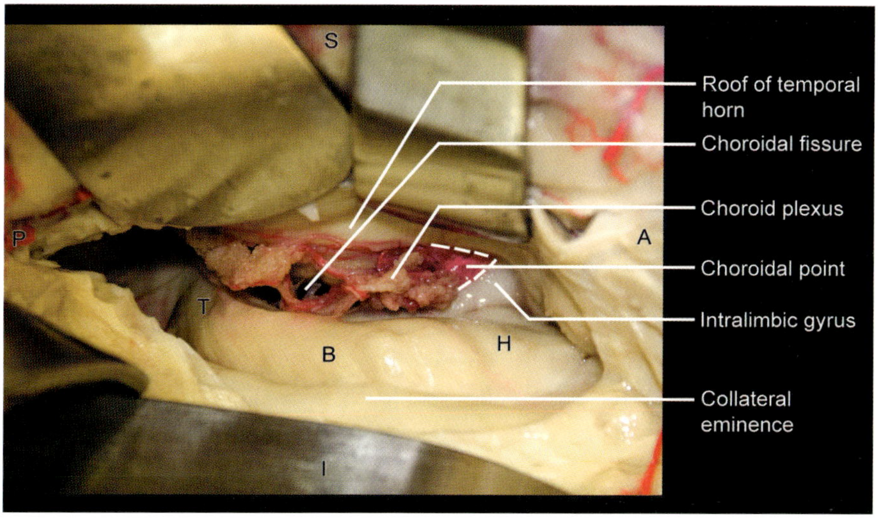

Fig. 2.12: Panoramic view of the right hippocampus. The middle temporal gyrus and subcortical white matter have been opened and retracted to expose the contents of the temporal horn of the lateral ventricle. The hippocampus is readily visible as a curved structure including the head (H), body (B), and tail (T). Note the small digitations on the hippocampal head. The choroid plexus and choroidal fissure which is open in this specimen are visible. The choroidal point marks the entry of the anterior choroidal artery in to the temporal horn and is the anterior most end of the choroidal fissure. The velum terminale forms a triangle (dashed lines) and immediately anterior to that is the infralimbic gyrus.
(A: Anterior; I: Inferior; P: Posterior; S: Superior).

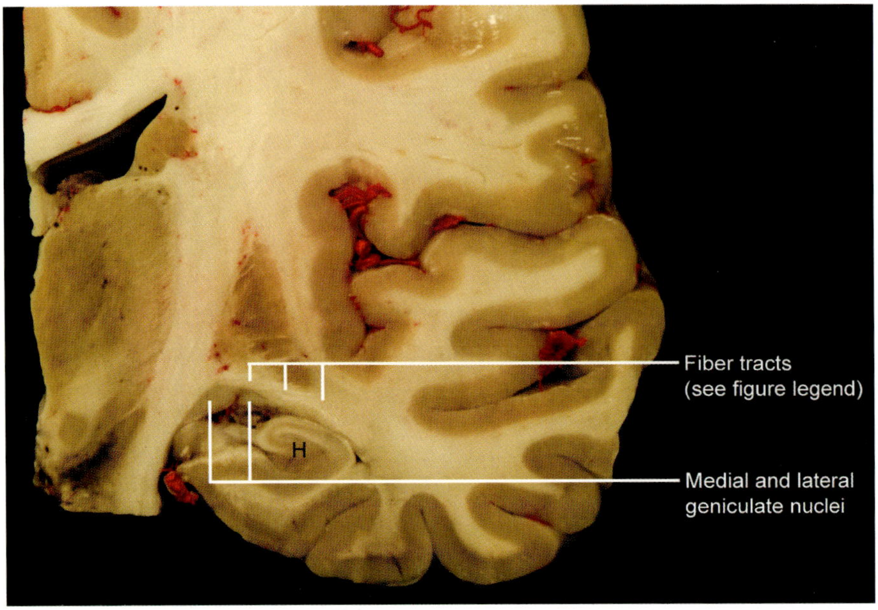

Fig. 2.13: Coronal cross-section of the left temporal lobe demonstrating the contents of the roof of the temporal horn. Anteriorly the roof is part of the temporal stem followed by the optic radiation fibers as one marches posteriorly. Further posterior, the roof is composed of various traversing fibers including the parietopontine, occipitopontine, occipitocollicular, and occipitotectal fibers. Also, the medial and lateral geniculate bodies form the superomedial roof the temporal horn and are considered as part of the roof.

geon to the location of the surrounding anatomy due to its consistent anatomical relationships. Anteriorly, the choroidal fissure begins posterior to the choroidal point and can be identified by following the choroid plexus to its attachment. The choroidal fissure is associated with the body and tail of the hippocampus; the head is associated with the uncus. Posteriorly, the choroidal fissure is intimately associated with the mesial pia of the temporal horn. Opening the fissure and pia leads to the ambient cistern and thalamus, structures that need to be handled with high regard.

Vascular Relationships of the Temporal Lobe (Fig. 2.14)

Internal Carotid Artery

The supraclinoid segment of the carotid artery is closely related to the uncus. It bifurcates to the anterior and middle cerebral arteries at the medial end of the Sylvian fissure and the anterior part of the uncus.

Posterior Communicating Artery

The posterior communicating artery (PCom) is the first branch of the supraclinoid internal carotid artery (ICA). It arises in the posteromedial or posterolateral part of the ICA and has an entirely cisternal course. Although it is not directly in communication with the mesial temporal lobe, the PCom and its perforators are visible during mesial temporal lobe resection.

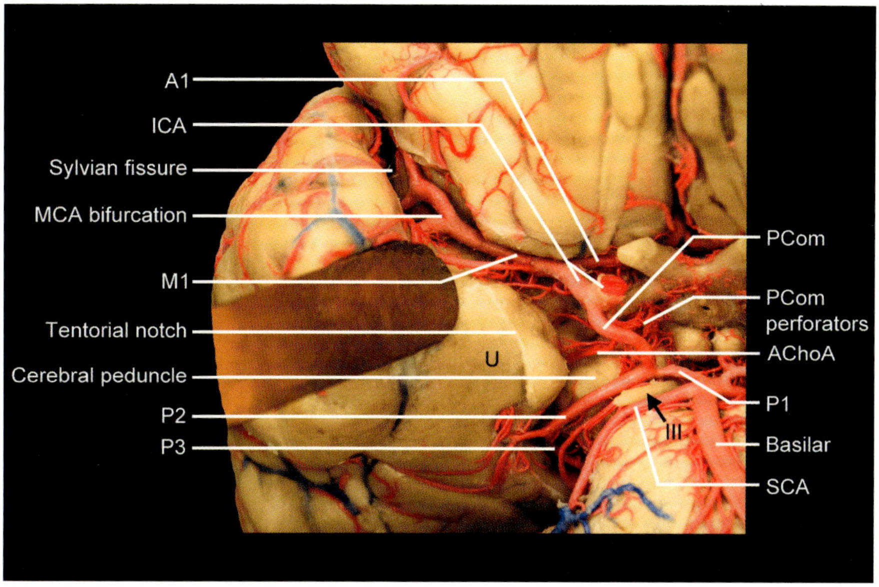

Fig. 2.14: Basal view of the right hemisphere demonstrating the vascular anatomy and relevant relationships. The supraclinoid segment of the internal carotid artery (ICA) is medial to the uncus and bifurcates to the A1 segment of the anterior cerebral artery and the M1 segment of the middle cerebral artery at the anterior superior part of the uncus. The posterior communicating artery (PCom) is the first branch of the ICA with many perforators that are visible during mesial temporal lobe surgery. The anterior choroidal artery (AChoA) is the second branch of the ICA which runs on the medial surface of the uncus along the posterior edge of the infralimbic gyrus before entering through the choroidal point and supplying the choroid plexus of temporal horn. The P1 segment of the posterior cerebral artery (PCA) is visible along with its branches supplying the parahippocampal gyrus. The P2 and P3 segments are visible wrapping around the cerebral peduncle. The P2 segment of the PCA and its perforators are intimately related to the mesial hippocampal sulcus. (U: Uncus; III: Cranial nerve 3; SCA: Superior cerebellar artery)

Anterior Choroidal Artery

The anterior choroidal artery (AChoA) arises distal to the PCom from the ICA off of the posterolateral wall in most instances. The artery runs in the carotid and crural cisterns respectively, medial to the uncus. It passes the posterior edge of the infralimbic gyrus to enter the temporal horn of the lateral ventricle. The entry of the AChoA to the temporal horn and its relationship to the choroidal point and choroidal fissure is constant and serves as a crucial surgical landmark for the neurosurgeon's orientation.

Posterior Cerebral Artery

The posterior cerebral artery (PCA) is the terminal branch of the basilar artery and is composed of four segments. P1 is the segment from the bifurcation to the PCom. The P2 segment extends from the PCom and wraps around the crus cerebri and midbrain. P3 begins at the posterior midbrain and runs in the quadrigeminal cistern, ending at the calcarine fissure. P4 is the cortical segment.

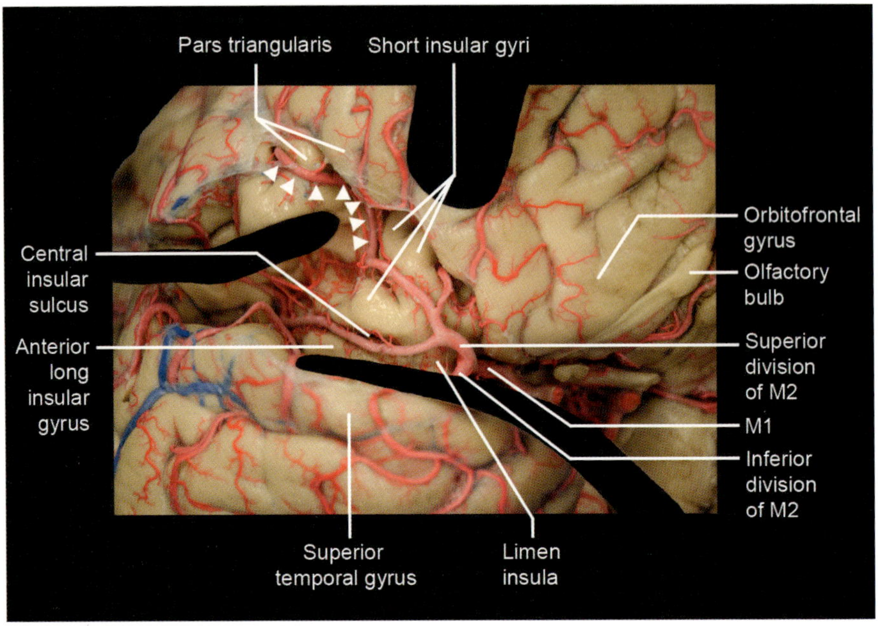

Fig. 2.15: View of the right Sylvian fissure divided in order to visualize the MCA, divisions, and the surrounding anatomy. M1 bifurcation is usually at or just distal to the limen insula as seen. The superior division often divides into branches that run across the insula. The superior branch, as it approaches the superior insular sulcus, turns over the apex of the insula immediately below the triangular cistern (arrowheads) and its branches run in the horizontal and vertical rami of the triangular cistern as they reach the frontal operculum.

The P2 segment of the PCA travels around the crus cerebri and midbrain and, as such, has an intimate relationship with the posterior uncus and the hippocampal sulcus. The medial and lateral posterior choroidal arteries and the hippocampal arteries arise from the P1 and P2 segments of the PCA. The hippocampal arteries enter the hippocampus by penetrating the dentate gyrus, the fibriodentate sulcus, and the hippocampal sulcus. The hippocampal arteries can also partly or fully originate from the anterior choroidal artery (Uchimura artery).

Middle Cerebral Artery

The middle cerebral artery (MCA) arises from the bifurcation of the ICA and is divided into four segments (Fig. 2.15). The M1 segment is from the bifurcation to the limen insula. M2 is the segment from the limen insula to the temporal operculum and includes all the branches related to the insula. The M3 segment is from the temporal operculum to the cortex and includes all the branches related to the temporal, frontal and parietal lobes. The M1 segment is spatially related to the uncus and serves as an important landmark during mesial resection of the amygdala. Because of the lack of a clear anatomical boundary between the superomedial amygdala and the basal ganglia, the proximal M1, when viewed through the mesial pia of the uncus, serves as a limiting landmark for superior extent of resection. Moving ahead, the proximal M1 gives off the lenticulostriate branches from its posterior superior surface starting as early as the

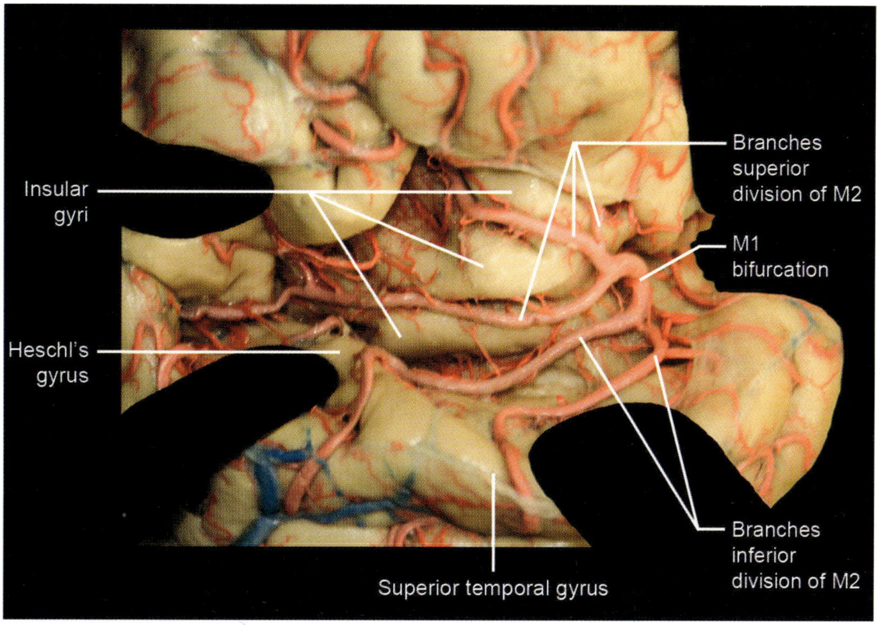

Fig. 2.16: Right Sylvian fissure dissected with attention to the inferior division of the M2 branches. The inferior division branch runs across the inferior insular sulcus before turning laterally over the surface of Heschl's gyrus and exiting the fissure.

carotid bifurcation and extending within 1.5 cm of the limen insula. In most cases, the MCA bifurcates immediately distal to the limen insula.

The inferior branch runs in the inferior circular sulcus (Fig. 2.16) and it can be readily identified during dissection. The superior branch of the MCA has a more convoluted route and deserves special care during dissection. As it approaches the superior insular sulcus, the superior branch of the MCA "turns" over the apex of the insula immediately below the triangular cistern and its branches run in the horizontal and vertical sulci of the triangular cistern as they reach the frontal operculum.

INSULA

The insula is a cortical structure that is completely encased by the frontal, parietal, and temporal opercula and only becomes visible when the Sylvian fissure is divided. Functions of the insula have been attributed to memory, effect, autonomic control, gustation, and olfaction. However, the true comprehensive function of the insula remains unknown.

The insula has been described as a pyramid-shaped structure with its apex pointing downward. Three distinct sulci define the boundaries of the insula: the superior, inferior, and anterior limiting sulci. The surface anatomy of the insula (Fig. 2.17), when the Sylvian fissure is divided widely, presents a large lateral and a smaller anterior surface. The lateral surface has intimate connections with the frontal and parietal operculi superiorly and the temporal operculum inferiorly. It is divided by a prominent central sulcus into a larger anterior and a smaller

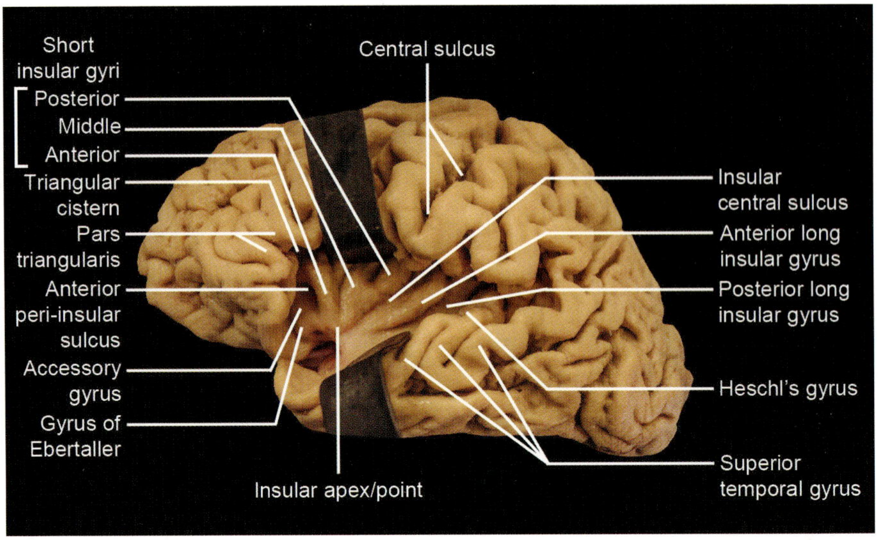

Fig. 2.17: The left hemisphere with retraction of Sylvian fissure exposing the insular surface. The lateral surface of the insula is intimately associated with the frontal and temporal opercula. The central insular sulcus divides it into the larger anterior and smaller posterior zones. The anterior zone is composed of the anterior, middle, and posterior short gyri. The posterior zone consists of the long anterior and posterior gyri. All gyri converge at the insular point/apex. As noted in this figure, the central sulcus of the insula correlates with the central sulcus of the frontal lobe. The anterior surface of the insula is composed of the vertically oriented accessory gyrus and a smaller horizontal gyrus of Ebertaller.

posterior zone. The anterior zone is composed of the anterior, middle, and posterior short gyri that converge at the insular apex; an anatomical landmark that correlates with the triangular cistern of the frontal operculum on the cerebral surface. The posterior zone of the lateral surface of the insula consists of the long anterior and posterior gyri.

The central sulcus of the insula correlates anatomically with the Rolandic fissure or central sulcus that divides the frontal and parietal lobes (Fig. 2.17). Given the hidden nature of the insula on surface anatomy during surgery, this consistent landmark can help identify the location of the insular central sulcus.

The anterior surface of the insula is composed of a vertical accessory gyrus and the short transverse gyrus of Ebertaller. Both gyri converge at the insular pole or apex. The medial border of the anterior surface of the insula is the anterior limiting sulcus. The anterior insular cleft is the space between the anterior surface of the insula and the posterior and lateral orbital gyri.

The medial border of the insula has close relationships with the central deep nuclei and fiber tracks of the frontoparietal lobes. The superomedial limit of the anterior limiting sulcus of the insula is related to the anterior limb of the internal capsule and the frontal horn is reached just deep to that (Fig. 2.18). The body of the lateral ventricle is located medial to the superior limiting sulcus. The caudate and putamen are located medial to the body of the insula (Fig. 2.19). Anteriorly, the caudate is associated with the middle short gyrus and, posteriorly, the body and tail of putamen are medial to the posterior long gyrus of the insula. The internal capsule is medial to the caudate and putamen along the central portion of the body of insula.

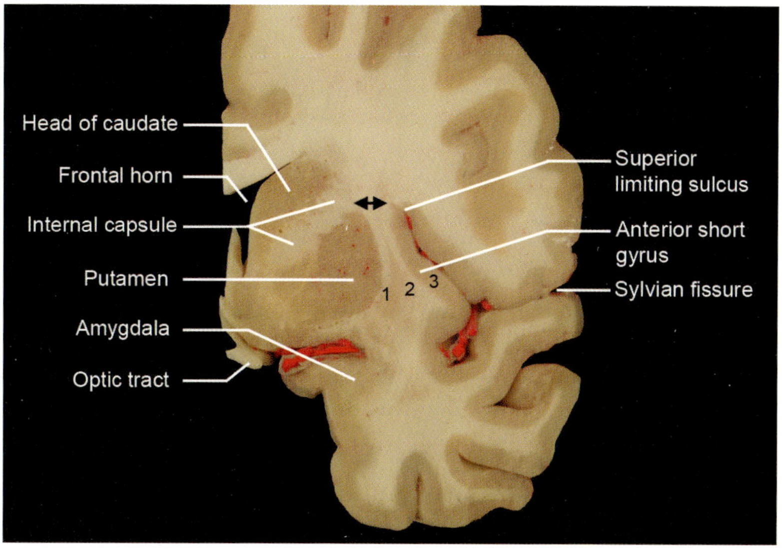

Fig. 2.18: Coronal cross-section of the left hemisphere at the level of anterior insula corresponding to the anterior short gyrus. The proximity of the superior limiting sulcus to the internal capsule is demonstrated by the double arrowheads. The anterior short gyrus abuts the extreme capsule (3), followed by the claustrum (2), external capsule (1), and the putamen.

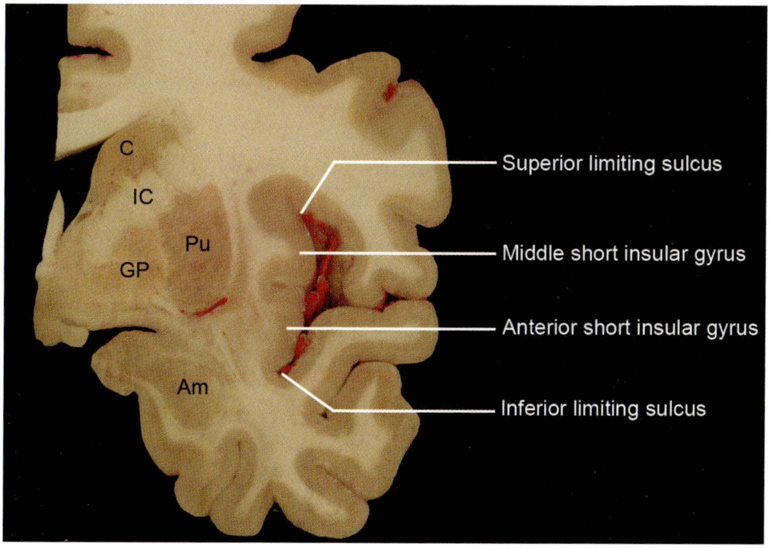

Fig. 2.19: Coronal cross-section of the same specimen as in Figure 2.18, at the level of the body of insula corresponding to the middle short gyrus. Note the internal capsule is now farther away from the mesial border of the insula, separated by the putamen and globus pallidus. The superior limiting sulcus is a consistent landmark that corresponds to the superior border of putamen medially. The interior limiting sulcus of the insula corresponds to the superior portion of the amygdala.
(Am: Amygdala; C: Caudate; IC: Internal capsule; GP: Globus pallidus; Pu: Putamen).

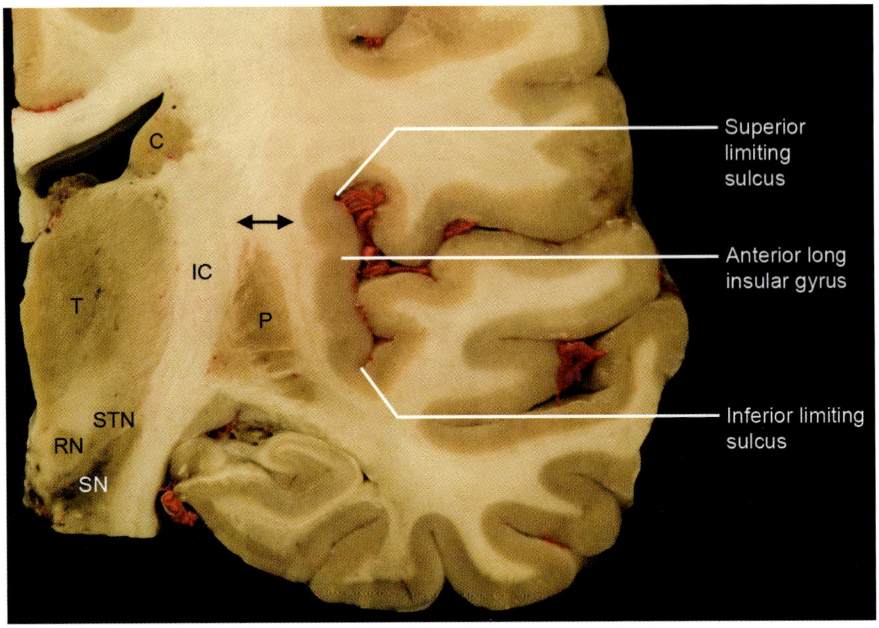

Fig. 2.20: Cross-section of the same specimen as in Figures 2.18 and 2.19, further posteriorly at the level of the anterior long insular gyrus. Note the decrease in size of the putamen and globus pallidus and direct proximity of the anterior long insular gyrus to the capsule fibers (double arrowhead).
(C: Caudate; IC: Internal capsule; P: Putamen; RN: Red nucleus; SN: Substantia nigra; STN: Subthalamic nucleus; T: Thalamus).

The extreme anterior and posterior limits of the internal capsule, however, are directly medial to the insula with no "protective layer" of basal ganglia and, hence, vulnerable to insult during surgery (Figs. 2.18 and 2.20).

SYLVIAN FISSURE AND OPERCULAR ANATOMY

The sylvian fissure arachnoid separates the frontoparietal operculum from the temporal operculum. The anterior arachnoid of the fissure bridges the anterior portion of the planum polare of the temporal lobe to the posterior portion of the lateral, posterior, and medial orbital gyri and merges with the arachnoid of the carotid and chiasmatic cisterns. The sylvian fissure is anatomically separated from the carotid cistern by the limen insula. The arachnoid membrane of the sylvian fissure is also continuous with the arachnoid surface of the anterior surface of the insula. The planum polare of the temporal lobe, which is anterior to Heschl's gyrus, correlates with the precentral gyrus, pars opercularis, and pars triangularis of the frontal operculum (Fig. 2.21). From there, the planum polare turns medial, forms the temporal pole, and ends at the rhinal sulcus that separates it from the uncus.

At the point of the triangular cistern of the frontal operculum, the sylvian fissure divides into three rami: (1) the horizontal, (2) anterior ascending and (3) posterior (Fig. 2.21). The anterior horizontal ramus of the Sylvian fissure separates the pars orbitalis from the pars trian-

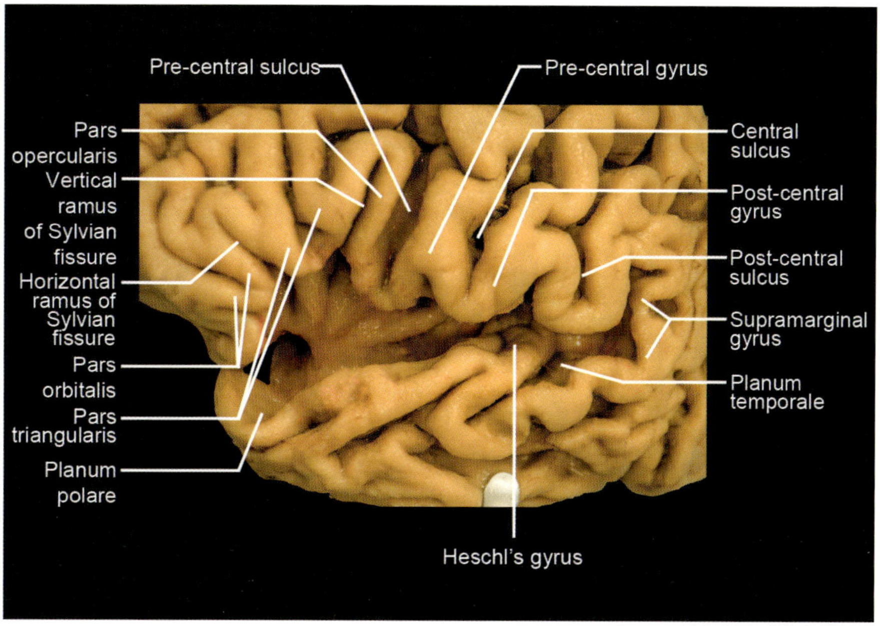

Fig. 2.21: Left hemisphere surface anatomy of the perisylvian region demonstrating the frontal and temporal opercular structures and their corresponding relationships. The planum polare of the temporal lobe corresponds with the pars triangularis, pars orbitalis, and the precentral gyrus. The Sylvian fissure divides anteriorly to the vertical and horizontal rami as shown. Posteriorly, the Sylvian fissure ends by forming the superior and inferior rami of the supramarginal gyrus. The postcentral gyrus of the parietal lobe corresponds anatomically with Heschl's gyrus and is a consistent landmark for its identification.

gularis of the frontal operculum and continues medially as the anterior limiting sulcus of the insula. The anterior ascending ramus delineates the border of the pars triangularis. The posterior ramus is the longest one and is directed posteriorly and superiorly, ending at the supramarginal gyrus. As one marches posteriorly, the postcentral gyrus of the parietal operculum and Heschl's gyrus on the temporal operculum correlate anatomically in the Sylvian fissure.

CHAPTER

3

Approaches to the Mesial Temporal Lobe for Epilepsy

Sepehr Sani, Joshua T Wewel, Richard W Byrne

INTRODUCTION

This chapter will provide an overview of surgery involving the anterior temporal lobe and mesial limbic structures. The unique nature of this operation as opposed to tumor surgery is the "normal" anatomy that is encountered. Therefore, a thorough understanding of the anatomical structures and their inter-relationships in the mesial temporal lobe is essential to obtaining consistently safe surgical results.

The original temporal lobectomy was reported by Dr Penfield at the Montreal Neurological Institute. Since then the technique has been standardized via a lateral approach with additional "selective" approaches and transsylvian approaches described subsequently, careful preoperative work-up is imperative in identifying the seizure focus. Patients suspected of having temporal lobe seizures are evaluated by electroencephalography (EEG) and video EEG studies as well as high-resolution magnetic resonance imaging (MRI), single-photon emission computed tomography (SPECT), SPECT coregistered to MRI (SISCOM), and magnetic encephalography (MEG) studies to pin point the ictal focus. If there is uncertainty, invasive epidural or subdural grids and electrodes, or depth electrodes can be placed for prolonged monitoring. Once the focus is identified and surgery ensues, intraoperative electrocorticography (ECoG) before, during, and after resection can be employed to confirm cessation of abnormal spikes.

At the authors' institution, a tailored temporal lobectomy approach is employed where the lateral neocortical resection is customized to each patient's condition. This is followed by amygdalohippocampectomy including the body of the hippocampus to the level of the ambient cistern.

SURGICAL ANATOMY

A detailed anatomical review of the temporal lobe has been provided in the previous chapter. As it pertains to the surgical procedure, the surface anatomy of the temporal lobe and the interrelationship of the mesial structures are reviewed here.

Starting at the sylvian fissure, the surface of temporal lobe is covered in a coronal plane by seven gyri which are divided respectively by seven sulci (Figs. 3.1A and B). The superior,

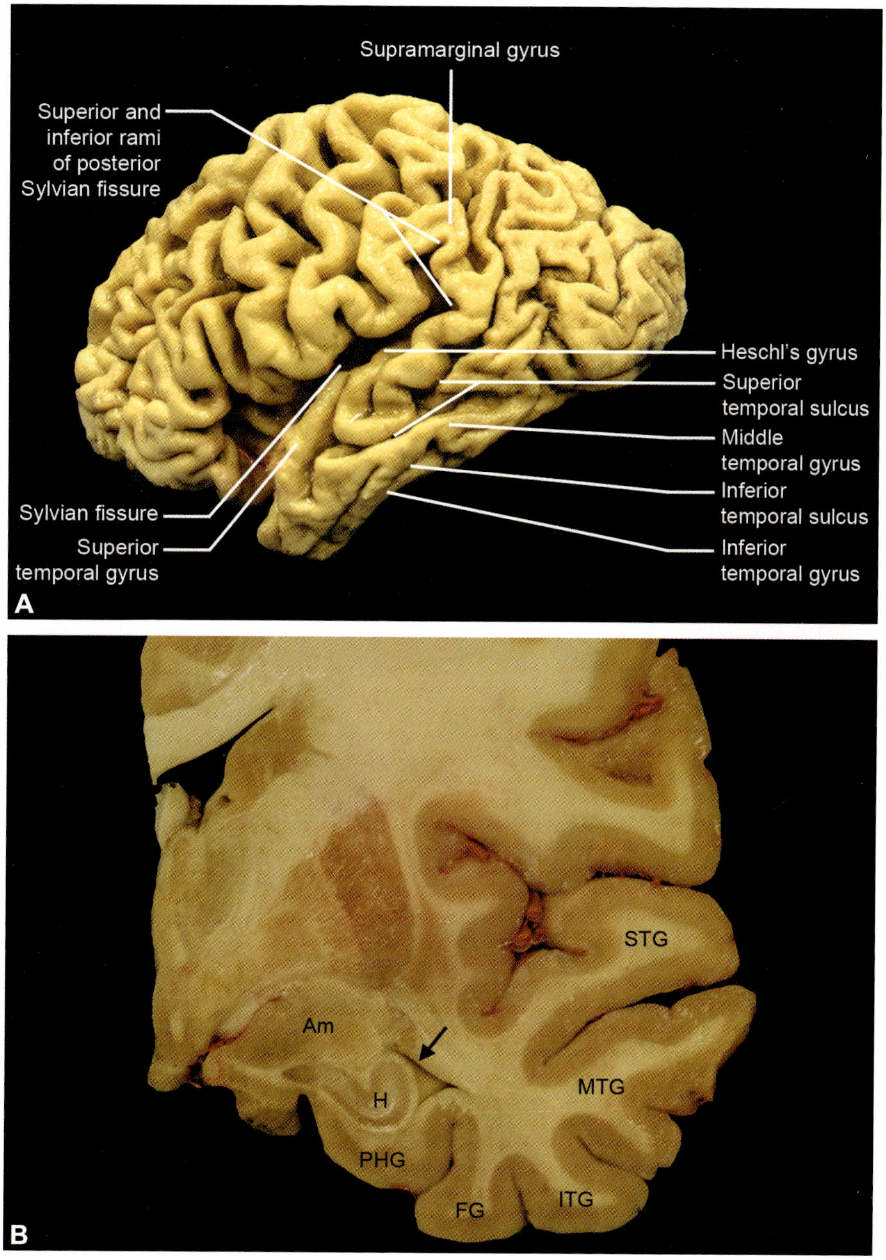

Figs. 3.1A and B: Surface anatomy of the temporal lobe. (A) Left hemispheric surface demonstrating the anatomy of the temporal lobe. The superior temporal gyrus may be interrupted by crossing sulci. Heschl's gyrus merges laterally with the superior temporal gyrus. (B) Cross-sectional anatomy of the left temporal lobe at the level of the amygdala and head of hippocampus. Arrow indicates temporal horn.
(Am: Amygdala; STG: Superior temporal gyrus; H: Hippocampus; MTG: Middle temporal gyrus; PHG: parahippocampal gyrus; FG: Fusiform gyrus; ITG: Inferior temporal gyrus).

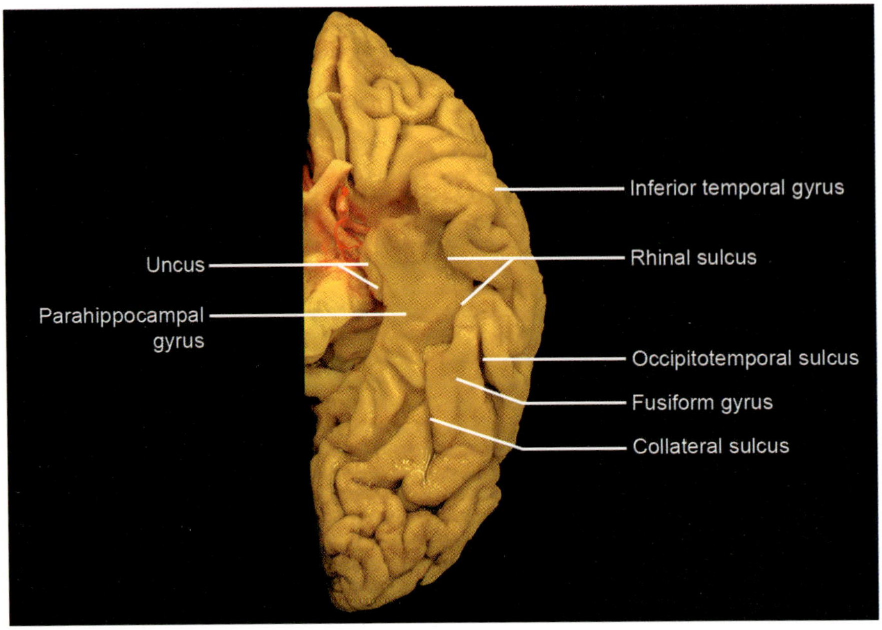

Fig. 3.2: Basal view of the left hemisphere demonstrating the surface anatomy of the basal and mesial temporal lobe.

middle, and part of the interior temporal gyrus occupy the lateral surface of the lobe. The superior temporal gyrus is consistently well demarcated and extends from the temporal pole posteriorly to becoming the posterior limb of the supramarginal gyrus. The middle temporal gyrus is more tortuous in its course and ends posteriorly as the posterior limb of the angular gyrus. The inferior temporal gyrus is inconsistent in its anteroposterior course and occupies the inferolateral angle of the lobe.

The fourth gyrus is the fusiform or occipitotemporal gyrus which runs from the temporal pole posteriorly to the occipital gyrus (Fig. 3.2). The medial border of the gyrus is marked by an extremely consistent and important landmark, the collateral sulcus, a deep and consistent sulcus. When viewed in the coronal orientation, the sulcus ends immediately ventrolateral to the temporal horn and can be used as a relative landmark in finding the temporal horn. The sulcus originates in the occipital lobe and extends anteriorly, ending before the rhinal sulcus of the uncus. The collateral sulcus will sometimes end in continuity with the rhinal sulcus.

The next gyrus is the parahippocampal gyrus which lies in the inferomedial part of the temporal lobe. It wraps around and is continuous with the hippocampus proper. Laterally, the parahippocampal gyrus is bordered by the collateral sulcus and on the medial side it is bordered by the ambient cistern. The parahippocampal gyrus bends anteriorly at the uncal sulcus. The uncal sulcus is continuous posteriorly with the hippocampal sulcus and contains the hippocampal arteries. Anteriorly, the parahippocampal gyrus ends at the rhinal sulcus which separates it from the temporal pole.

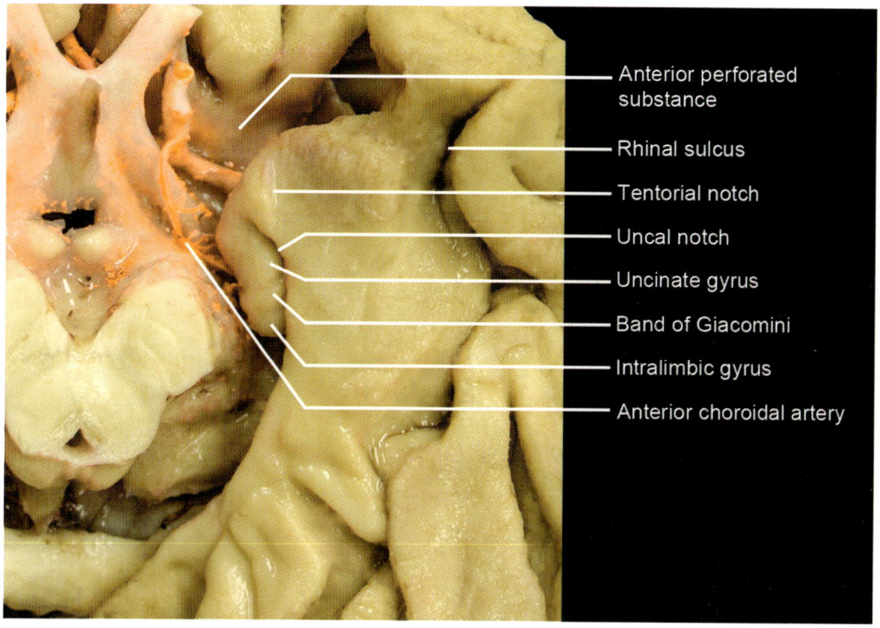

Fig. 3.3: Magnification of the left basal view demonstrating the anatomy of the uncal gyri and relevant vascular anatomy. The majority of the uncus is identified as the uncal gyrus. The uncal gyrus is immediately adjacent to the carotid artery, the posterior communicating artery, the anterior choroidal artery, with the third cranial nerve beneath. The superior aspect of the uncus largely consists of the amygdala and its connections to the hippocampus. The blood supply to the amygdala arises both from the anterior choroidal artery and from descending perforators from the middle cerebral artery. Immediately superior to the uncal gyrus lies the second gyrus of the uncus, the semilunar gyrus. This small gyrus marks the superior aspect of the uncus and runs in parallel to the endorhinal sulcus. Moving posteriorly, at the posterior medial aspect of the amygdala lies the intralimbic gyrus of the uncus. This small gyrus, which lies between the amygdala and the hippocampus along the crural cistern, is a critical surgical landmark. It is critical because the crural cistern is only a potential space, separating the mesial temporal structures from the crus cerebri of the midbrain by a single layer of arachnoid. This rectangular shaped landmark is crucial during surgery as it identifies a safe deep border of resection early on.

Anteriorly, the uncus can be thought of via its embryology as an anterior, mesial extension of the parahippocampal gyrus. The mesial rotation of the uncus brings it in contact with the contents of the carotid cistern. The majority of the uncus is identified as the uncal gyrus. The uncal gyrus is immediately adjacent to the carotid artery, the posterior communicating artery (PCOM), the anterior choroidal artery, with the 3rd cranial nerve beneath. The superior aspect of the uncus largely consists of the amygdala and its connections to the hippocampus. The blood supply to the amygdala arises both from the anterior choroidal artery and from descending perforators from the middle cerebral artery.

Immediately superior to the uncal gyrus lies the second gyrus of the uncus, the semilunar gyrus (Fig. 3.3). This small gyrus marks the superior aspect of the uncus and runs in parallel to the endorhinal. Directly superior to the endorhinal sulcus runs the optic tract which continues posteriorly to form the roof of the temporal horn beginning at the level of the choroidal point.

Moving posteriorly, at the posterior medial aspect of the amygdala lies the intralimbic gyrus of the uncus (Fig. 3.3). This small gyrus, which lies between the amygdala and the hippocampus along the crural cistern, is a critical surgical landmark. It is critical because the crural cistern is only a potential space, separating the mesial temporal structures from the crus cerebri of the midbrain by a single layer of arachnoid. This rectangular shaped landmark is crucial during surgery as it identifies a safe deep border of resection early on. Once identified as a roughly rectangular structure between the amygdala and hippocampus, just anterior to the choroidal point and the velum terminale, a subpial aspiration of this thin gray matter structure will quickly uncover the arachnoid separating the mesial temporal lobe from the brainstem.

Just posterior to the intralimbic gyrus is the velum terminale, the thin triangular shaped membrane that is formed by the fibers of the fimbria and stria terminalis (Fig. 3.4). This is also

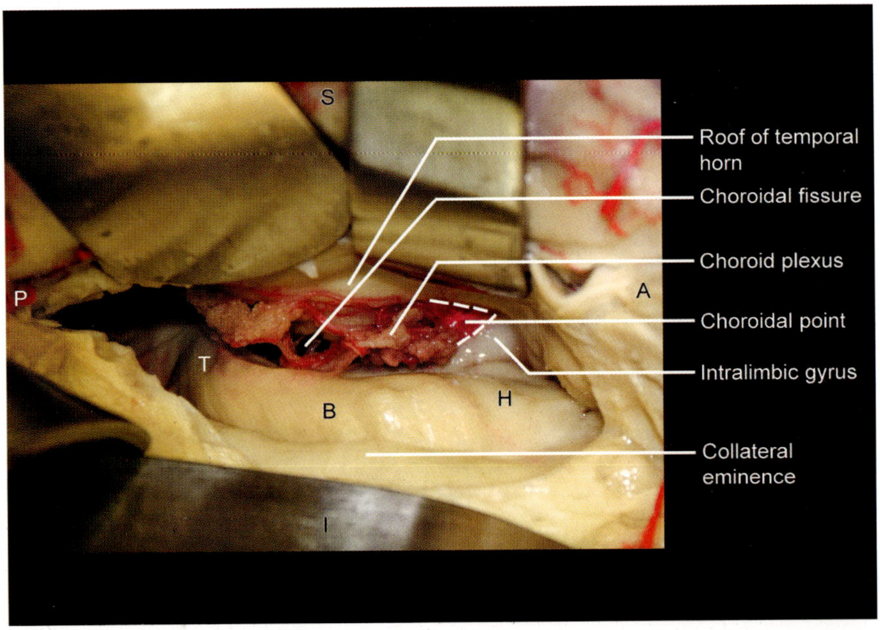

Fig. 3.4: Panoramic view of the right temporal horn demonstrating the structures of the mesial temporal lobe as viewed during surgery. The middle temporal gyrus has been opened and subcortical white matter dissected with retractors placed on the roof of temporal horn. When entering the temporal horn, the hippocampus is seen as a bulging structure with a crescent shape The hippocampal head is wide and approximately 15 mm in length (H), containing digitations on its surface. The body (B) of the hippocampus begins at the choroidal point and is approximately 10 mm in length before narrowing and blending posteriorly to the tail. The tail (T) wraps around the ambient cistern into the trigone of the ventricle. The dorsal border of the hippocampus is formed by the choroidal fissure, an important landmark. The intralimbic gyrus is a rectangular shaped structure that is identified immediately anterior to the velum terminale as shown. The velum terminale is a thin triangular shaped membrane that is formed by the fibers of the fimbria and stria terminalis. This is also known as the inferior choroidal point. Immediately posterior to this structure is the choroidal point, a thin pinkish colored membrane that is visible upon retraction of the choroid plexus. The choroidal point is an extremely consistent structure which marks the entry point of the anterior choroidal artery. Its identification is one of the first steps after entering the temporal horn (P: Posterior; S: Superior; A: Anterior; I: Inferior).

known as the inferior choroidal point. Immediately posterior to this structure is the choroidal point, a thin pinkish colored membrane that is visible upon retraction of the choroid plexus. This remarkably consistent anatomical structure is the entry point of the anterior choroidal artery. Its identification is one of the first steps after entering the temporal horn during surgery as it allows the surgeon orientation to adjacent anatomy stated earlier.

On the mesial side, moving posteriorly from the choroidal point, the hippocampus is the next visible structure. When entering the temporal horn, the hippocampus is seen as a bulging structure with a crescent shape (Fig. 3.4). The hippocampal head is wide and approximately 15 mm in length. The body of the hippocampus begins at the choroidal point and is approximately 1 cm in length before narrowing and blending posteriorly to the tail. The tail wraps around the ambient cistern into the trigone of the ventricle.

The dorsal border of the hippocampus is formed by the choroidal fissure, an important landmark. Mesially, the hippocampal sulcus is a potential space and usually adherent, containing multiple small vessels that need to be divided during resection. The internal wall is formed by the dentate gyrus and the outer wall is formed by the subiculum of the parahippocampal gyrus (Fig. 3.5).

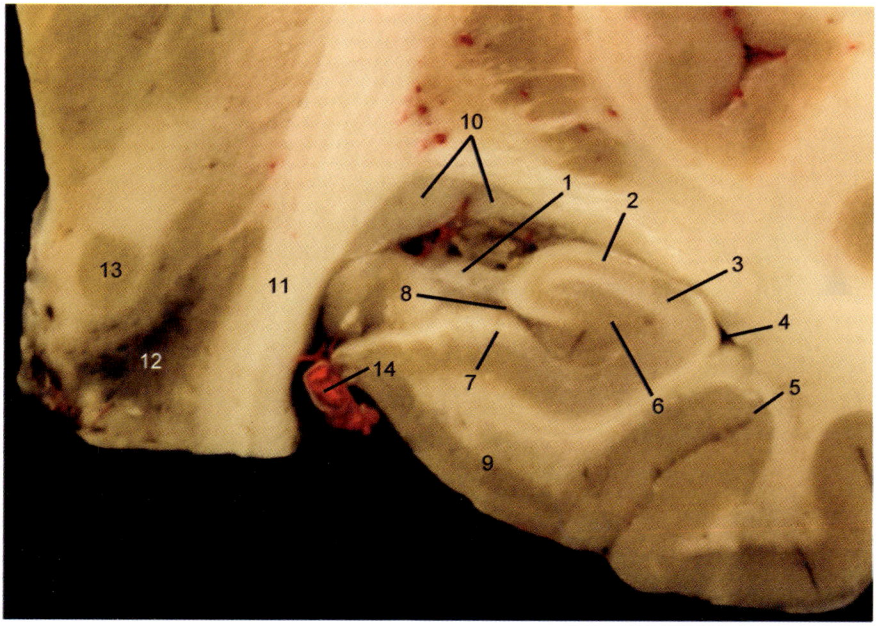

Fig. 3.5: Coronal cross-section of the left temporal lobe with magnification of the hippocampus anatomy. The lateral wall of the hippocampus is in the temporal horn (4). Note the relationship of the collateral sulcus (5) bulging into the temporal horn, the collateral eminence. Inferiorly, the hippocampus is surrounded by the parahippocampal gyrus (9). The hippocampus proper is composed of the dentate gyrus (6), CA4 and 3 regions, as well as the CA2 (2), and CA1 (3) regions. The hippocampal sulcus (8) divides the hippocampus from the parahippocampal gyrus. The fimbria and fornix (1) carry the outflow of information from the hippocampus. (1: Fornix; 2: CA2 region; 3: CA1 region; 4: Temporal horn; 5: Collateral sulcus; 6: Dentate gyrus; 7: Subiculum; 8: Hippocampal sulcus; 9: Parahippocampal gyrus; 10: Medial and lateral geniculate nuclei; 11: Cerebral peduncle; 12: Substantia nigra; 13: Red nucleus; 14: Posterior cerebral artery).

The fimbria is a narrow flat white band that runs along the internal border of the hippocampus just above the dentate gyrus (Fig. 3.5). It terminates anteriorly at the velum terminale. As the fimbria moves posteriorly it accumulates fiber tracks and eventually moves away from the hippocampus, forming the fornix proper.

OVERVIEW OF THE RELATIONSHIP BETWEEN THE MESIAL TEMPORAL LOBE, THE BASAL CISTERNS, AND THEIR CONTENTS

Uncus and Amygdala

Perhaps the biggest key to safe surgery in the mesial temporal lobe is acquiring a deep understanding of the relationship between mesial temporal lobe structures and the neighboring structures of the adjacent basal cisterns. This relationship should be fully understood and committed to memory prior to operating in the mesial temporal lobe. These relationships are entirely three dimensional, but are readily identifiable with careful identification of landmarks. The exception is the superior border of the amygdala with the basal ganglia, which is only identifiable by extrapolation.

Safe resection in this region is best achieved through subpial resection, preserving the deep mesial arachnoid whenever possible. This is almost always possible in amygdalohippocampectomy for epilepsy, usually possible in cases of low-grade glioma, and sometimes possible in high-grade gliomas. This is however, often not possible in vascular pathology, where proximal control requires dissection of the basal cistern vasculature. It should be remembered that the anterior choroidal artery may be single or duplicated, small or large. In some cases, a large portion of the blood supply to the internal capsule will come from large mammillary perforators arising from PCOM. These perforators should also be preserved. The superior aspect of the uncus largely consists of the amygdala and its connections to the hippocampus. The blood supply to the amygdala arises both from the anterior choroidal artery and from descending perforators from the middle cerebral artery.

Moving posteriorly, at the posterior medial aspect of the amygdala lies the third gyrus of the uncus, the intralimbic gyrus. This small gyrus, which lies between the amygdala and the hippocampus along the crural cistern, is a critical surgical landmark. It is critical because the crural cistern is only a potential space, separating the mesial temporal structures from the crus cerebri of the midbrain by a single layer of arachnoid. This very subtle transition between the mesial temporal lobe and the brainstem is essential to identify early in surgery in order to determine a safe deep border. Adding to this hazard is the fact that the anterior choroidal artery also runs in this space on its way to the choroidal point. This landmark is easily identified in epilepsy surgery, but may be difficult to identify in tumor and vascular cases. Once identified as a roughly rectangular structure between the amygdala and hippocampus, just anterior to the choroidal point and the velum terminale, a subpial aspiration of this thin gray matter structure will quickly uncover the arachnoid separating the mesial temporal lobe from the brainstem.

Just posterior to the intralimbic gyrus is the velum terminale, the thin membrane covering the entry of the anterior choroidal artery which enters the choroidal fissure to provide blood supply to the choroid plexus of the temporal horn.

The Hippocampus and the Choroidal Fissure

Embryologically, the hippocampus starts as a dorsal structure in mammals, and in most mammals it remains dorsal, with connections to the temporal lobe. In humans, the hippocampus migrates over time between the 10th and the 20th week in development. The result is the converse of the relationship that exists in many other mammals, with the dominant portion of the hippocampus lying in the mesial temporal lobe and preserved connections to the superior aspects of the limbic system via the cingulate gyrus, the fimbria-fornix, the indusium grisium, and the fasciolar gyrus. An understanding of this embryological connection is essential to a deeper understanding of limbic anatomy.

The term limbic at its root implies bordering. The structure of the limbic system borders is the diencephalon. In fact, the limbic structures, if disconnected at the superior aspect of the amygdala, could be completely dissected away from the diencephalon from the temporal pole to the descending columns of the fornix. This fact highlights the critical nature of the choroidal fissure as a surgical landmark. The choroidal fissure and its accompanying choroid plexus extend in a bent C-shaped from the choroidal point to the Foramen of Munro. The choroidal fissure begins at the choroidal point, a point that marks the transition between the pes hippocampus anteriorly and the hippocampal body. As such, the choroidal point is a reliable and useful landmark. Once the choroidal point is identified within the temporal horn it marks a midpoint of the temporal aspect of the mesial temporal limbic anatomy. A retractor placed at in the coronal plane of the choroidal point that elevates the roof of the temporal horn allows for a panoramic view of the surface anatomy of the temporal horn. Anterior to the choroidal point, velum terminale leads to the intralimbic gyrus. The amygdala is identified anterior-laterally as a gray structure swelling into the ventricle. The amygdala is thus the anterior-superior border of the temporal horn.

Posterior to the choroidal point, the roof of the ventricle must be respected surgically if the optic radiations are to be preserved. The only exception is the case where the surgical pathology has already irreversibly disconnected the optic radiations from the thalamus and the occipital pole. This requires a low entry into the ventricle during the exposure, or a transsylvian approach that enters anterolateral at the level of the choroidal point. Once the roof of the ventricle is identified and protected, it may be elevated to expose the rest of the ventricle. Any further opening of the ventricle posteriorly should be performed in an axial plane, as inferiorly as possible. An entry immediately lateral to the collateral sulcus is ideal. Meyer's loop projects laterally and anteriorly from the lateral geniculate body. In order to preserve the majority of these projections, a low and anterior opening into the ventricle is best. Although preservation of Meyer's loop is ideal, in reality, a complete disruption of Meyer's loop and the resultant superior quadrantanopia is not a particularly disabling problem. In fact, few patients notice the deficit, as it does not interfere with reading, working or driving.

Looking posteriorly in the temporal horn, the lateral geniculate body and its projections can be identified, as can be the lateral thalamus. A thin retractor applied gently to the roof of the temporal horn opens the ventricle to expose the atrium of the ventricle. At this level, the choroid plexus and the tail of the hippocampus can be seen bending superior-medially behind the pulvinar of the thalamus. From the anterior exposure, this is the most posterior extent of a safe resection of the hippocampus, and constitutes a radical hippocampectomy. From a posterior exposure, the choroid plexus and the fornix can be followed anteriorly above the thalamus in the lateral ventricle to the Foramen of Munro. This posterior exposure of the tail of the hippocampus can be achieved via a transmiddle temporal gyrus exposure, a subtemporal transcollateral exposure, an endoscopic posterior approach, or a posterior interhemispheric precuneus approach. Identifying the choroid plexus of the atrium and then following it anteriorly into the lateral ventricle above and the temporal horn anterior-inferior from the pulvinar is a reliable way to avoid injury to the thalamus in cases where the pathology obscures normal borders.

Resecting Pathology from the Junction of the Hippocampus/Parahippocampus and the Deep Mesial Basal Cisterns

Once the temporal horn has been entered and the regional anatomy has been identified, the target pathology can be addressed. In epilepsy surgery, resecting the hippocampus is done in a subpial plane. Whether the resection is done en bloc, or by transecting the hippocampus in a coronal plane is a matter of comfort for the surgeon. A transection in a coronal plane at the level of the choroidal point will naturally separate the hippocampus into the head anteriorly and the body posteriorly. The hippocampus can be separated from the amygdala at the level of the intralimbic gyrus anteriorly, and can be removed along with the parahippocampal gyrus by subpial aspiration in a sagittal plane just mesial to the collateral sulcus down to the basal middle fossa arachnoid. The hippocampus will then roll away from the inferior pial connections up to the hippocampal sulcus, a double sided fold of arachnoid entering the hippocampus running in an axial plane from anterior to posterior. The hippocampal sulcus is the final critical surgical landmark in resection of the hippocampus. The hippocampal sulcus runs parallel to the posterior cerebral artery (PCA) and contains PCA perforators along its length that must be coagulated and divided. This vascular disconnection is the most important step in separating the mesial temporal structures from the basal cisterns. Although ventricular veins will drain into the basal vein of Rosenthal, they rarely pose a challenge in controlling. The exception to this is the highly vascular mesial temporal tumor or arteriovenous malformation (AVM). In these cases, controlling the *basal vein* is essential.

Occasionally, less common vascular configurations will be encountered. Variations in which a high riding superior cerebellar artery comes into the field may be identified on coronal MRI views before surgery. Also, it is not uncommon for the PCA to have a major branch displaced laterally underneath the parahippocampal gyrus. This also can be identified preoperatively and preserved, if it is not entangled with the surgical pathology. Finally, the 4th cranial nerve runs the length of the mesial temporal lobe just underneath the incisura.

If the incisura must be incised in order to improve surgical exposure, the 4th cranial nerve should be identified and preserved. Overly aggressive coagulation along the incisura should also be avoided.

ANTERIOR TEMPORAL LOBECTOMY WITH AMYGDALOHIPPOCAMPECTOMY

Although the term anterior temporal lobectomy refers to the resection of all neocortical structures of the anterior temporal lobe, in reality a tailored approach is more common. The extent of lateral neocortical resection is determined on a case by case basis and depends on several factors including electrocorticographic (ECoG), functional imaging, and vascular anatomic findings. At the author's institution a combination of data are used to determine the extent of resection along each of the lateral temporal gyri.

Positioning and Equipment

The patient is placed in the lateral position and the head is fixated in pins. The head of the table is raised 20° to assist with venous drainage and the nose is elevated 20° above the horizontal sagittal plane to better visualize the long-axis of the hippocampus.

At the authors' institution, resection of mesial structures is performed using microscopic magnification and an ultrasonic aspirator for subpial dissection. Use of neuronavigation is optional, allowing the surgeon confirmation of anatomy (3.1 and 3.2). Subdural grids and strips as well as depth electrodes are made available for intraoperative ECoG.

A standard frontotemporal curvilinear incision is employed; the posterior margin of which being no further back than posterior margin of pinna to prevent necrosis. Soft tissue dissection is carried down until the root of the zygoma is visualized, marking the floor of the middle fossa. The scalp and temporalis muscle are reflected anteriorly. A standard frontotemporal craniotomy is performed. Bony resection is extended along the anterior temporal lobe using a rongeur in order to enhance visualization. The dura is subsequently opened and reflected anteriorly.

Baseline ECoG activity can be recorded at this time by placing a grid over the frontotemporal surface for neocortical structures. Generally, it is possible to slide a subdural strip around the base of the temporal lobe in the coronal place with the tip sitting on the medial parahippocampal gyrus. Placement of a depth electrode in the hippocampus through the middle temporal gyrus can be done. Anatomically, the electrode is inserted perpendicular to the surface of brain at the level of the middle temporal gyrus to a depth of 4 cm. Alternatively, stereotactic image-guided placement of depth electrodes can be employed.

Neocortical Resection

Neocortical resection generally extends between 3 cm and 4.5 cm from the temporal tip along the sylvian fissure on the dominant side, and between 3 cm and 5 cm on the nondominant side.

This may be altered by cortical stimulation mapping. However, important landmarks need to be identified and considered in customizing the resection. The vein of Labbe is usually identified on preoperative MRI and is confirmed intraoperatively. Attention is also paid to cortical M3 branches overlying superior and middle temporal gyri. Some arteries arise anteriorly only to curve posteriorly beyond the limits of resection and should be preserved.

Resection is done by subpial emptying of cortical and subcortical structures sequentially starting with the superior temporal gyrus or middle temporal gyrus (Figs. 3.6A to D). In many tailored resections, the superior temporal gyrus is spared as shown in Figure 3.6A. The resection is done using bipolar electrocautery or the ultrasonic aspirator. The superior temporal sulcus is identified and coagulated after confirmation of arterial end-branches. Dissection and aspiration continues inferomedially through the white matter until the collateral sulcus is identified. Once identified, attention is now turned back to the cortical pial incision line. The cortical resection now continues by subpial emptying of the middle and inferior temporal gyri as well as the fusiform gyrus. The medial wall of the fusiform gyrus is the collateral sulcus which has already been identified and is now joined. The posterior and medial margins of the lateral resection are now complete. To complete the en bloc resection of the neocortex, the dissection continues along the white matter temporal stem in the anterior direction at a 45° angle in order to avoid entering the ventricle. The collateral sulcus is a useful landmark; dissection generally should remain lateral and above this structure.

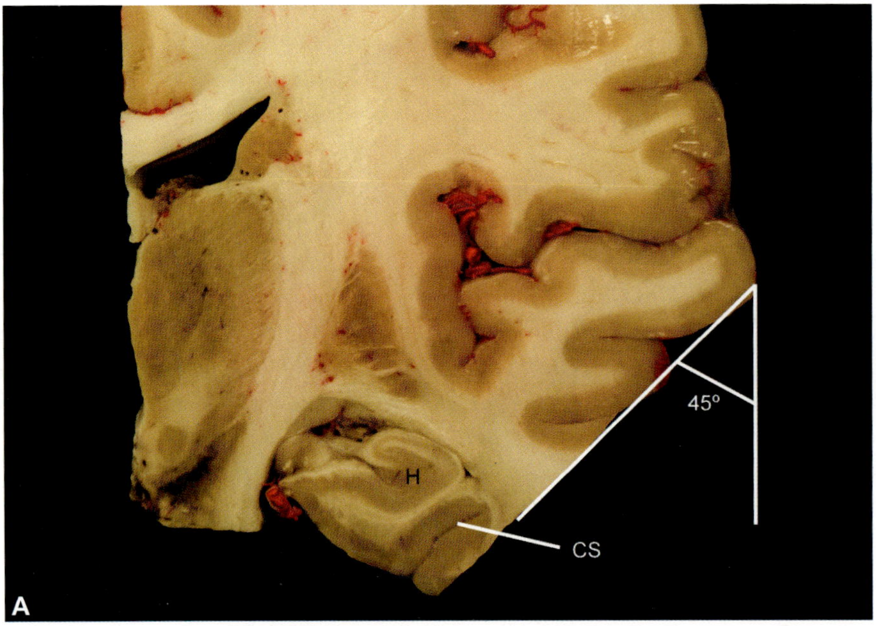

Fig. 3.6A: Cross-sectional demonstration of sequential removal of neocortical and mesial structures during anterior temporal lobectomy. (A) The middle and interior temporal gyrus are removed along with the fusiform gyrus. The dissection of the white matter is carried at an angle of 45° as shown to complete the lateral neocortical resection (H: Hippocampus; CS: Collateral sulcus).

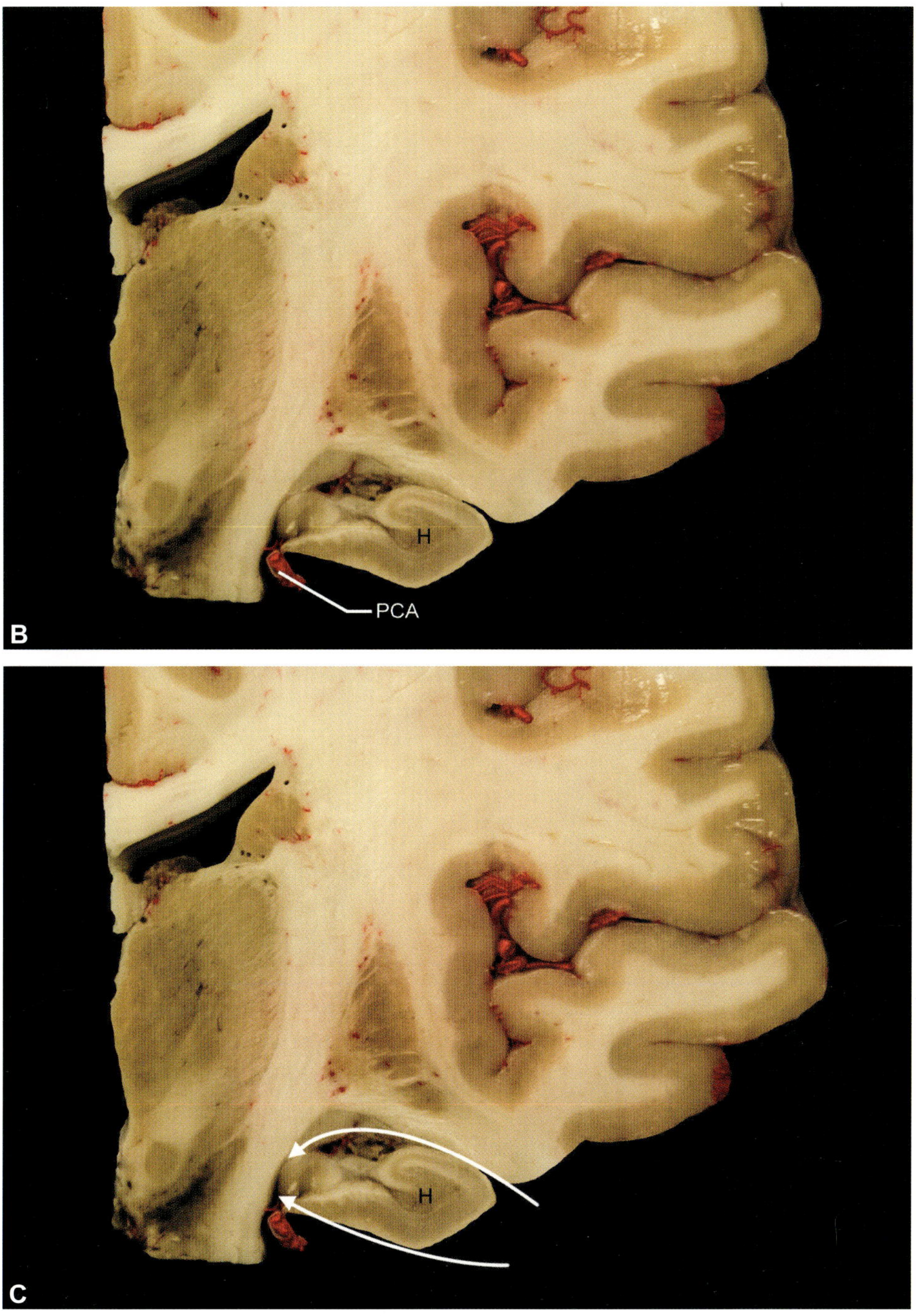

Figs. 3.6B and C: Next the temporal horn is identified and entered. The parahippocampal gyrus is now removed as shown. This allows the "rolling" of the hippocampus into the cavity of the resected parahippocampal gyrus, exposing the hippocampal sulcus an allowing for meticulous mesial division of perforator arteries as demonstrated by arrows in C (H: Hippocampus; PCA: Posterior cerebral artery).

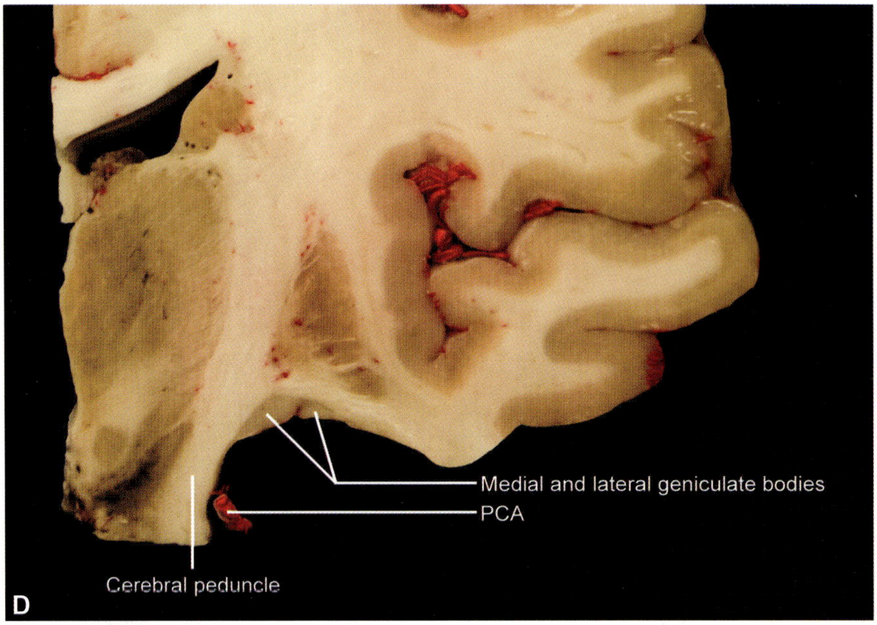

Fig. 3.6D: The hippocampus has been resected. Transpial view of the superior and mesial structures including the PCA, cerebral peduncle, and the geniculate nuclei.
(PCA: Posterior cerebral artery).

Resection of Uncus and Amygdala

For detailed illustration please see Figures 3.7A to L. The uncal gyrus makes up the majority of the anterior uncus. Using the microscope and ultrasonic aspirator (set at 30% of maximum suction and intensity) the uncal gyrus is emptied. Care must be taken to identify and preserve the mesial pial as it is reached. The next gyrus is the semilunar gyrus which marks the anterosuperior aspect of the uncus and runs parallel to the endorhinal sulcus. The anterior choroidal artery runs in this sulcus and can be seen through the pia during dissection. Immediately above the endorhinal sulcus lie the anterior most fibers of the optic radiation and thus it is imperative to avoid resection above the anatomic line of endorhinal sulcus.

As mesial resection continues, the carotid artery can be identified through the pia along with the 3rd cranial nerve. Further posterior, the free edge of the tentorium is identified through the pia. By preserving the mesial pia and using the M1 as the superior margin of aspiration allows the surgeon to radically resect the uncus safely. Visualization of proximal M1 through the mesial pia marks the anterosuperior line of resection of the amygdala. Further resection of the amygdala is done after the identification of the posterior-superior point.

Attention is now turned to the posterior resection line and the collateral sulcus. Dissection continues superior to the sulcus in the medial direction until the temporal horn is identified and entered. Next a nerve hook is used and the lateral ventricular wall is opened posteriorly. Two retractors are placed; one on the roof of the temporal horn to elevate it and to protect the fibers of

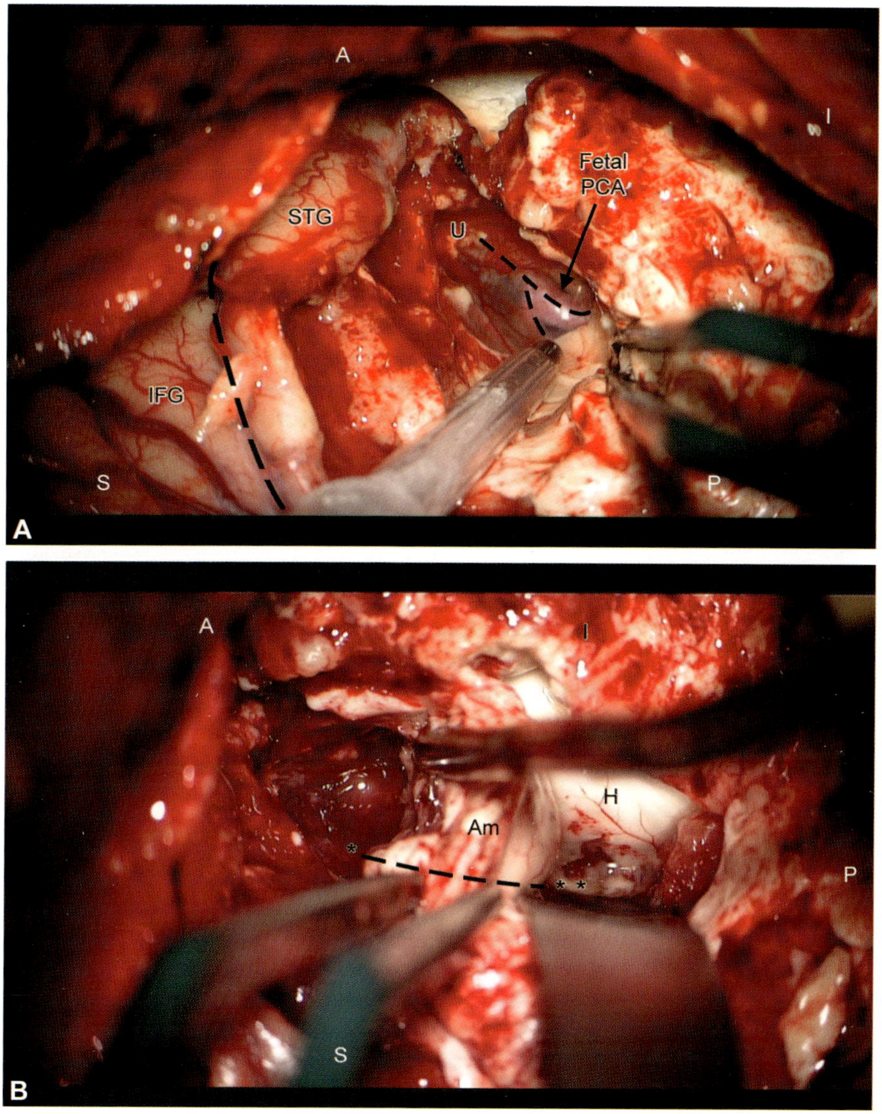

Figs. 3.7A and B: Intraoperative photographs demonstrating the sequential surgical steps of amygdalohippocampectomy. A right sided resection is shown. Neocortical resection has been completed. (A) Defining the anterosuperior border of amygdala resection. The sylvian fissure (dotted line), inferior frontal gyrus (IFG) and partially removed superior temporal gyrus (STG) are seen. The mesial pia is now visible after complete resection of the anterior uncus (U). The M1 segment is visible through the pia, which marks the anterosuperior border of the resection. Once identified, the location is marked and attention is now turned to the temporal horn further posteriorly. (B) A panoramic view including the temporal horn with a retractor placed along the roof to protect the contents including the fibers of the optic radiation. The hippocampal head (H) is visible. Once choroidal point and velum terminale are identified, the intralimbic gyrus is readily identifiable as the next anterior anatomical structure. The intralimbic gyrus is aspirated subpially (**). This marks the posterosuperior border of amygdala resection and also serves as a medial landmark during amygdala resection. A line drawn (dotted line) from the intralimbic gyrus (**) to the location of M1 (*) is demonstrated by the bipolar forceps as the resection line for the amygdala (A: Anterior; I: Inferior; P: Posterior; S: Superior).

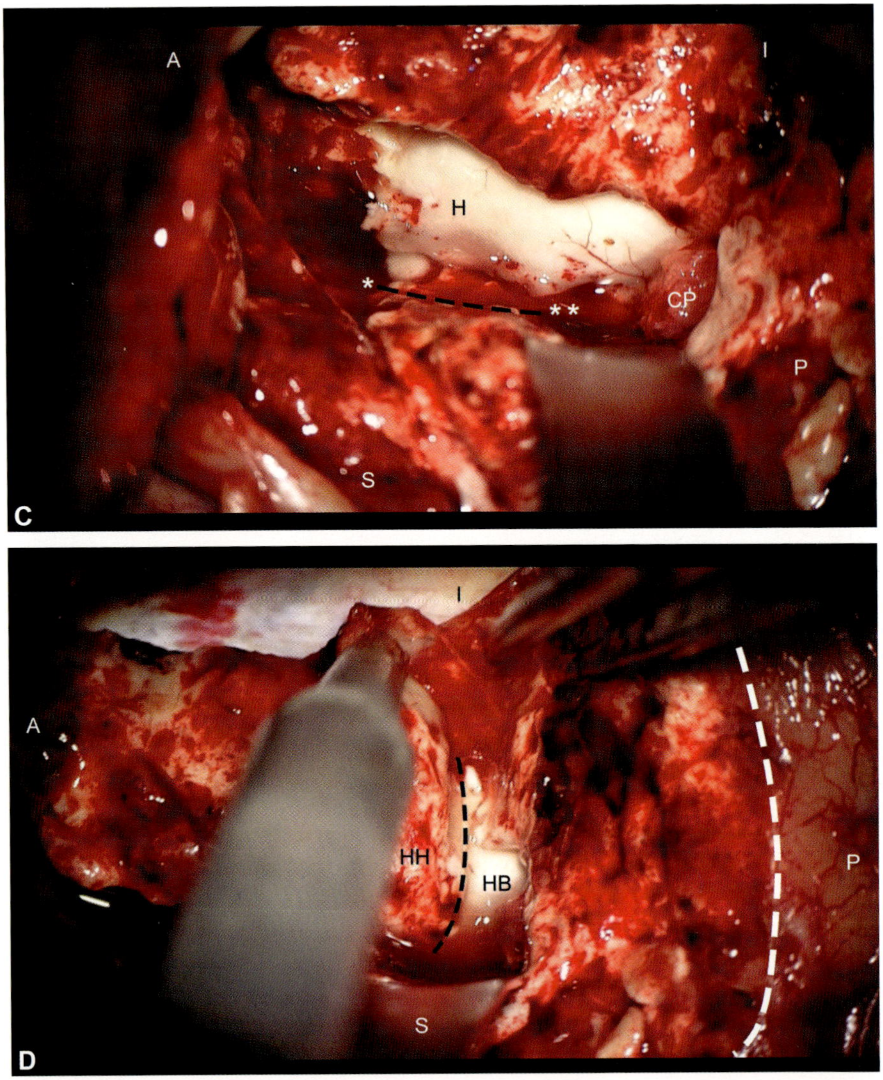

Figs. 3.7C and D: (C) The same view as B after resection of amygdala. The head of the hippocampus (H) is now' readily visible. A line drawn (dotted line) from the resected location of the intralimbic gyrus (*) to the location of M1 (**) is demonstrated. (D) Attention is now turned more posteriorly in order to resect the hippocampal head. Superficially, the posterior extent of neocortical resection is shown (white dotted line). Intraventricularly, the hippocampus head (HH) is severed (black dotted line) in the coronal plane from the body (HB) (CP: Choroid plexus; A: Anterior; I: Inferior; S: Superior; P: Posterior)

the optic radiation; the second thinner retractor placed and inserted in the temporal horn in the posterior direction parallel to the long-axis of the hippocampus to enhance visualization.

Inside the temporal horn, the choroid plexus is readily visible. It is carefully reflected and followed anteriorly to its beginning, which is the choroidal point. Once identified, the surgeon can immediately and safely navigate the surrounding anatomy. Immediately anterior to the

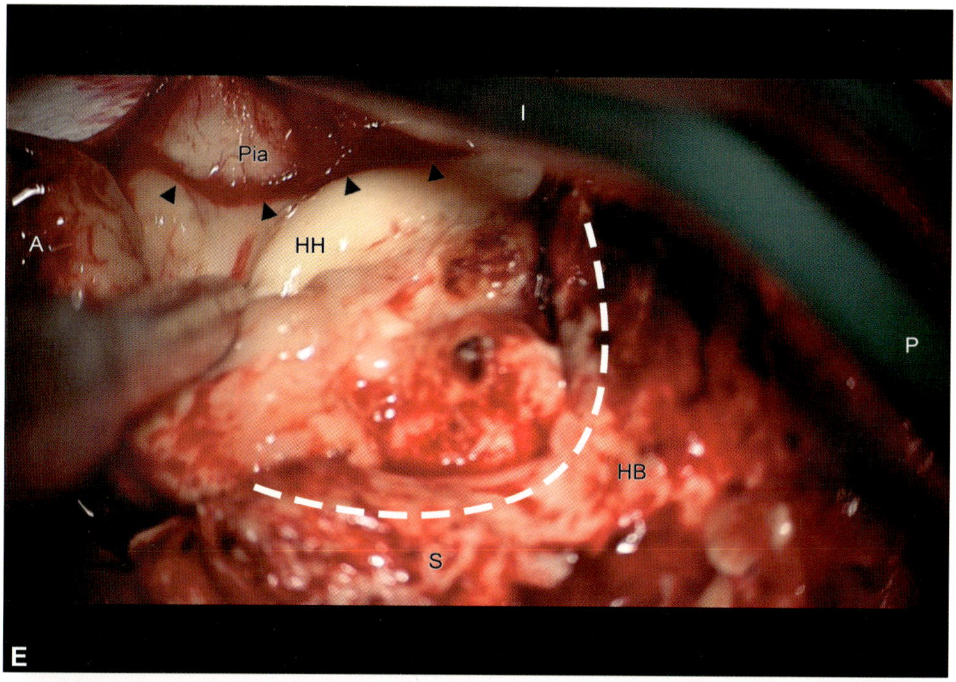

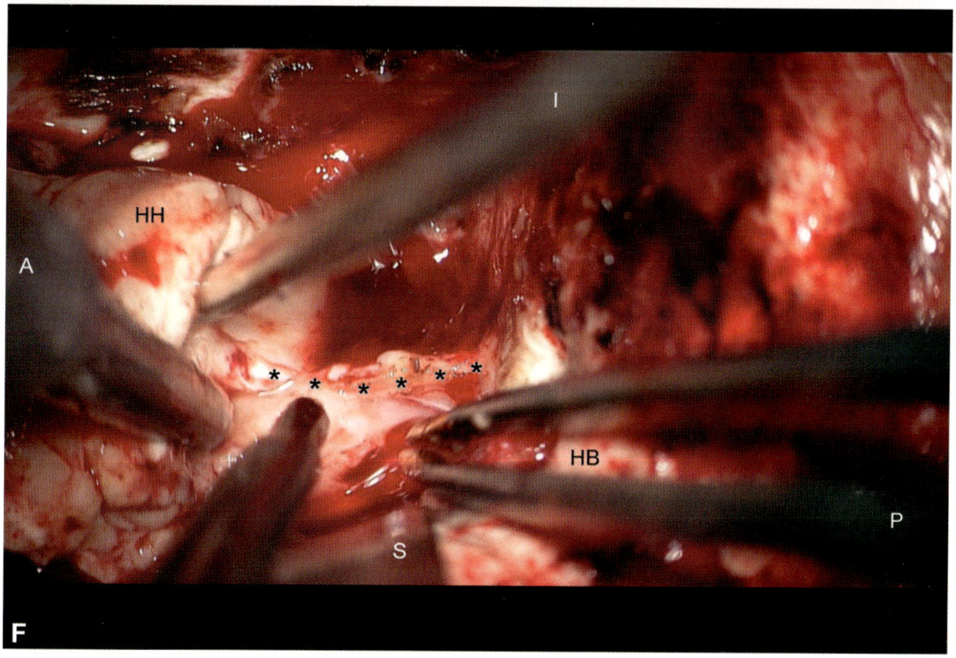

Figs. 3.7E and F: (E) Next the HH is laterally peeled off the pia (arrowheads). The coronal resection line and the hippocampus body (HB) are visible. (F) Attention is now turned to the medial side of the HH where the hippocampal sulcus (*) is identified and carefully coagulated and divided along the long-axis of the hippocampus. This step leads to complete separation of the HH (HH: Hippocampus head; HB: Hippocampus body; A: Anterior; P: Posterior; S: Superior; I: Inferior).

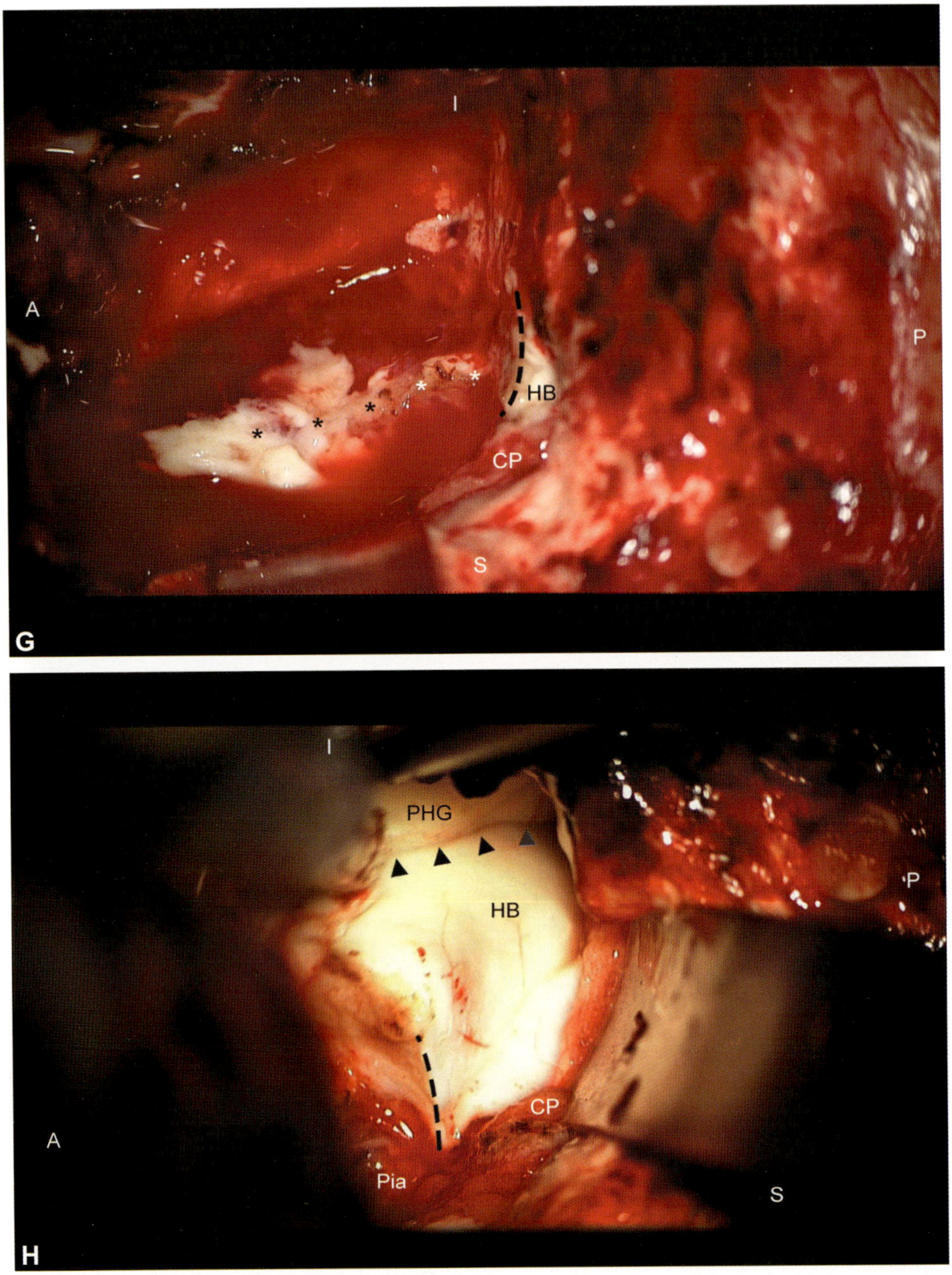

Figs. 3.7G and H: (G) The resection cavity after removal of the HH. The hippocampal sulcus remnant (*) and mesial pia are seen. (H) Now attention is turned posteriorly and the retractor is adjusted along the axis of the temporal horn to remove the hippocampus body (HB). In this view, the collateral eminence (arrowheads) and the remainder of the parahippocampal gyrus (PHG) are seen. The dotted line shows the coronal resection line of the body from the now removed HH (CP: Choroid plexus; A: Anterior; S: Superior; I: Inferior; P: Posterior).

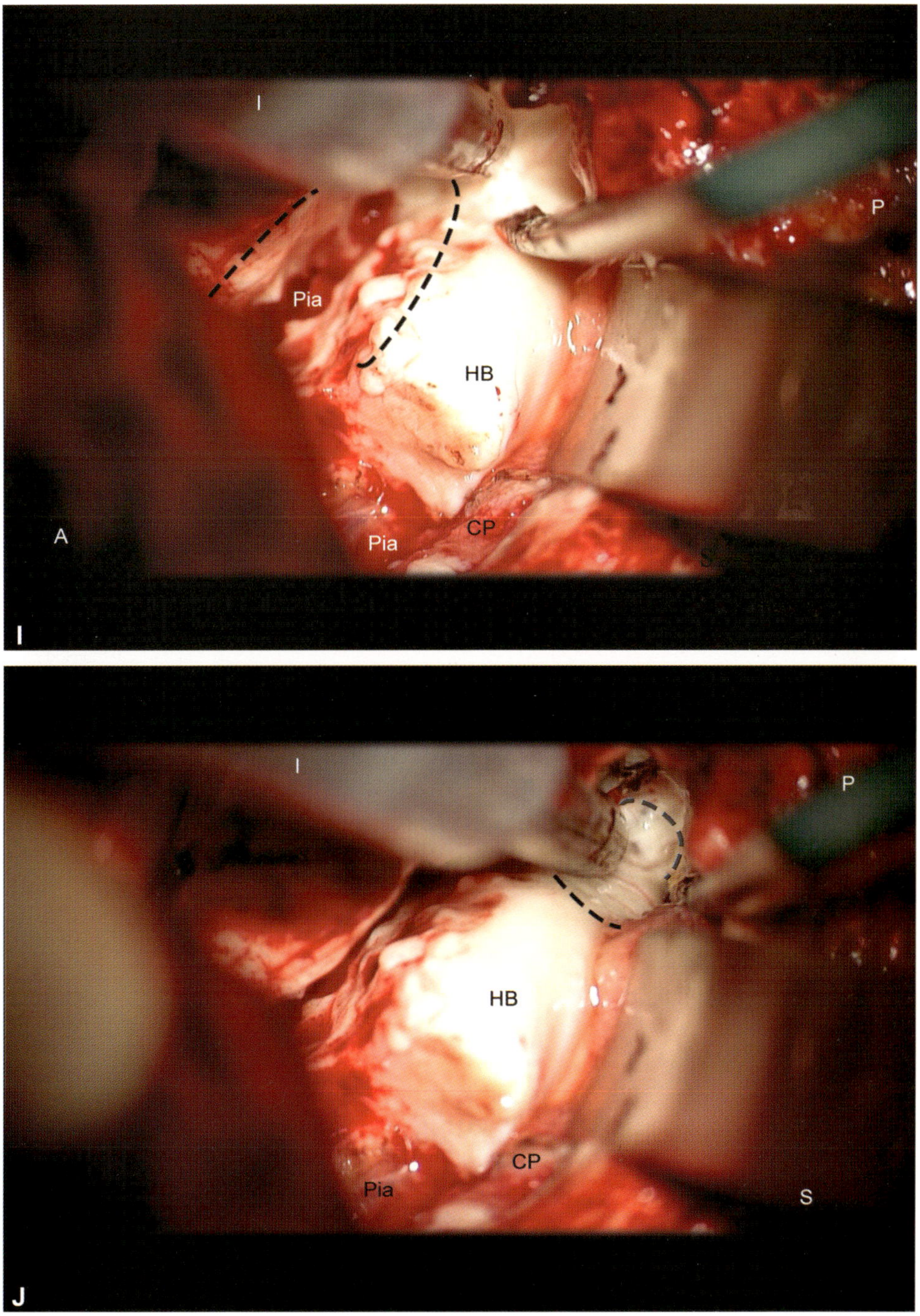

Figs. 3.7I and J: (I) The HB is first separated subpially on the lateral side (black dotted lines). (J) Next the HB is severed from the tail by aspiration as shown (black dotted lines) (HB: Hippocampus body; CP: Choroid plexus; A: Anterior; P: Posterior; I: Inferior; S: Superior).

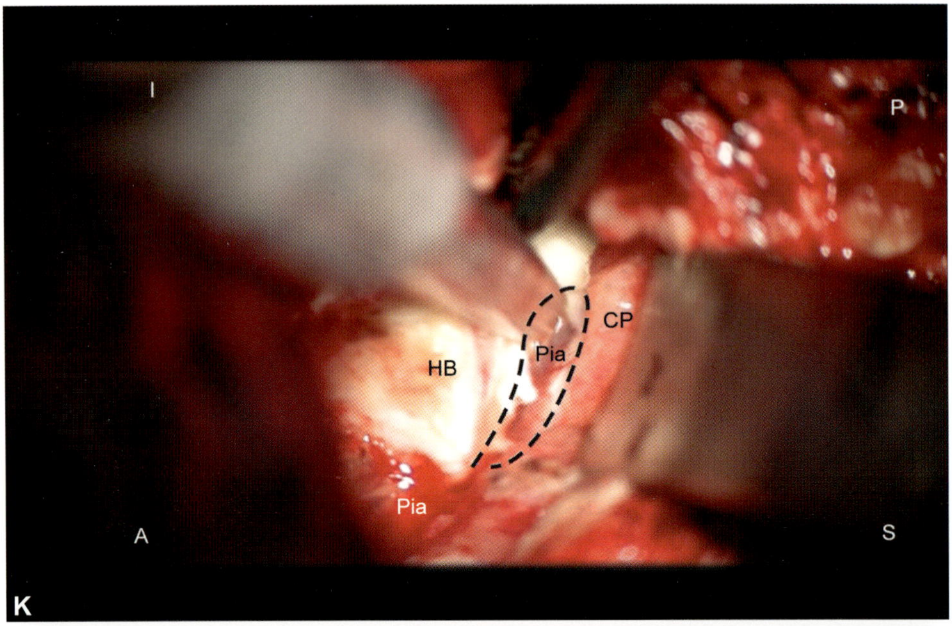

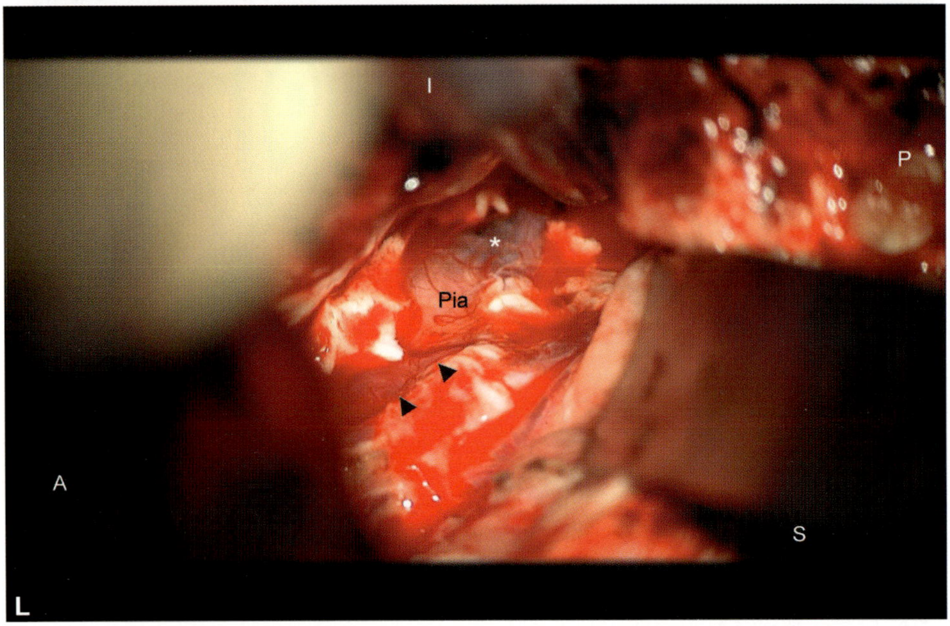

Figs. 3.7K and L: (K) Lastly, attention is turned medially. The hippocampal sulcus is identified, coagulated, and divided along the axis of the HB (black dotted lines) allowing its complete removal. (L) After removal of the HB, the medial pia is visible. The ambient cistern (*) and the posterior cerebral artery (arrowheads) can be seen through the pia.

(A: Anterior; P: Posterior; S: Superior; I: Inferior; CP: Choroid plexus; HB: Hippocampus body).

choroidal point is the velum terminale, a triangular structure. Anterior to the velum is a white rectangle which is the intralimbic gyrus of the uncus. This is the most posterior and superior gyrus of the uncus and is intimately associated with the cerebral peduncle medially. Ultrasonic aspiration of the intralimbic gyrus ensues with extreme care in order to identify the mesial pia which separates it from the peduncle. Once identified, the surgeon has a safe medial boundary identified.

The mesial pia of the intralimbic gyrus also marks the posterosuperior margin of safe amygdala resection. The superior limit of amygdala resection is now identified by an imaginary line drawn from the mesial pia of the intralimbic gyrus to the pia of the proximal M1 identified earlier. Subpial aspiration along this line continues caudally to completion. This allows for a radical yet safe anatomical resection of uncus and caudal amygdala.

Resection of the Hippocampus

The first step in the resection of the hippocampus involves the aspiration of the parahippocampal gyrus and subiculum, lateral to medial, starting at the medial side of the collateral sulcus (Figs. 3.6A to D). Care is taken to preserve the pia. As aspiration advances, the edge of the tentorium, the ambient cistern, and the posterior cerebral artery are exposed subpially.

Attention is now turned to the hippocampus. Aspiration of the parahippocampal gyrus allows the surgeon to physically rotate the hippocampus in the inferolateral direction, in the cavity of the parahippocampal gyrus (Figs. 3.6 to 3.8). This enhances the visualization of the fimbria medially. The hippocampus proper is then transected by aspirating the fimbria and dentate gyrus which exposes the hippocampal sulcus and the branches of the hippocampal artery entering the hippocampus. Meticulous attention is paid in identifying, coagulating and dividing the relevant branches while preserving the bypassing branches of the PCA in the vicinity. Transection of the hippocampal vasculature and sulcus ensues in an anterior to posterior direction, allowing the hippocampus head, body and desired amount of tail to be rolled and removed en bloc.

Occasionally, less common vascular configurations will be encountered. Variations in which a high riding superior cerebellar artery comes into the field may be identified on coronal MRI views before surgery. Also, it is not uncommon for the PCA to have a major branch displaced laterally underneath the parahippocampal gyrus. This also can be identified preoperatively and preserved, if it is not entangled with the surgical pathology.

SELECTIVE AMYGDALOHIPPOCAMPECTOMY

The selective approach to resection of the mesial temporal structures preserves the neocortical temporal lobe structures. This surgical variation can be employed in cases of mesial temporal pathology. It is debatable whether preservation of anterior temporal neocortex makes a difference in the overall outcome.

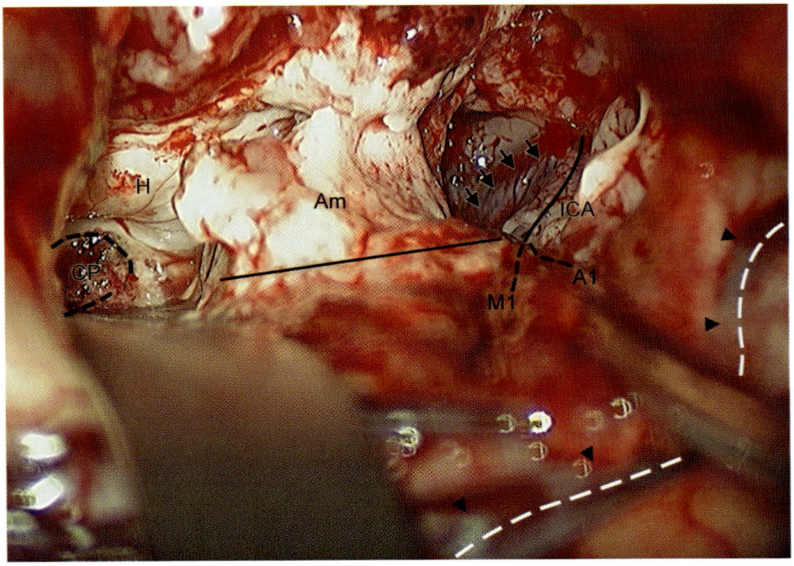

Fig. 3.8: Intraoperative photograph of a left sided approach to resection of mesial temporal structure. In this panoramic view, anatomic structures and their relationships for safe resection of the amygdala are shown. Superficially, the sylvian fissure (black dotted line) and sylvian vein (arrowheads) are seen. Anteriorly and deeper, the uncus has been largely removed and the medial pia is visible. The internal carotid artery (ICA), and its bifurcation (M1, A1) are visible. The anterior choroidal artery is seen (small arrows) traveling along the groove of the now removed rhinal sulcus to the choroidal point (CP). Posteriorly, the retractor is placed along the roof of the temporal horn, visualizing the choroidal point and velum terminale (dotted line). The cerebral peduncle is visible through the medial pia of the intralimbic gyrus. A line drawn (black solid line) from here to M1 marks the superior resection line of the amygdala (Am) (H: Hippocampus).

For this procedure, a more focused incision is made along the temporal area, centered on the middle temporal gyrus. After opening the dura, the cortical entrance is through the middle temporal gyrus at approximately 3 cm from the temporal pole. Dissection is carried medially in the white matter perpendicular to the cortical surface until the temporal horn is reached. Once opened, retractors are placed in the ventricle as described previously in the anterior temporal lobectomy section. Once panoramic view of the ventricular structures is obtained mesial resection is carried out.

During selective resection early transpial identification of M1 as the superior-anterior border of amygdala resection is not possible, different landmarks are used to carry out resection of the amygdala and uncus. The uncus is removed to the level of the anterior projection of the choroidal fissure.

Once the choroidal point, velum terminale, and intralimbic gyrus are identified, ultrasonic aspiration of the intralimbic gyrus and early identification of the mesial pia overlying the cerebral peduncle is performed. A useful landmark here paralleling the superior resection line of the amygdala is the anterior choroidal artery that can be followed from the choroidal point forward to the endorhinal sulcus. As resection continues anteriorly the endorhinal sulcus becomes the superior extent of resection. This way, the amygdala and uncus can be safely removed including all mesial intracisternal portions of the uncus.

Resection of the hippocampus subsequently ensues as previously described in the section on *anterior temporal lobectomy.*

TRANSSYLVIAN APPROACH TO AMYGDALOHIPPOCAMPECTOMY

The transsylvian-transcisternal approach to the mesial temporal structures is well described. For this approach, in order to improve visualization, following a standard frontotemporal craniotomy, the sphenoid wing and the orbital roof are made smooth by drilling. This is followed by dural opening and subarachnoid dissection of the sylvian fissure. The middle cerebral artery is identified and followed down to its origin and the arachnoid of the carotid cistern is sharply divided. The sylvian vein is followed anteriorly and managed. Attempts should be made at preserving the vein particularly, if preoperative imaging and intraoperative visualization suggest a dominant nature. Subsequently, the anterior temporal lobe is mobilized to allow visualization of the anterior choroidal (AChA) and posterior communication (PCoA) arteries. The AChA acts as a landmark that can be followed towards the inferior choroidal point. As visualization of the AChA around the uncus is lost, subpial dissection of the endorhinal sulcus may be required to visualize the inferior choroidal point. The parahippocampal gyrus can then be visualized with its superior boarders of the hippocampal sulcus and hippocampal formation. Medially the PCoA, AChA, and oculomotor nerve can be visualized. Selective amygdalohippocampectomy is carried out by incising the border of the hippocampus and uncal recess. The posterior margin of resection is limited by the lateral geniculate body or P2 bifurcation, superiorly by the optic tract, and laterally by the margin of the hippocampus at the collateral sulcus/eminence.

Advantages of the transsylvian approach include proximal control or all arterial vasculature. A clear advantage of acquiring access via the transsylvian route is eliminating cortical trauma via the transcortical or subtemporal approaches towards the mesial temporal lobe. Although it is advised to limit or eliminate the use of temporal lobe retraction, it is possible to sustain a retraction injury when visualization of the mesial temporal and perimesencephalic structures is limited, but necessary. A transsylvian-transcisternal approach for amygdalohippocampectomy has been described in efforts to spare the anterior optic radiations, however, visualization of the choroidal fissure can prove challenging. Although minimized, there is risk to the optic tract, optic radiations (Meyer's loop), and the oculomotor nerve.

Tumor Resection in the Anterior Temporal Lobe

The decision of which surgical approach one should take to mesial temporal limbic pathology is made after careful consideration of several factors. These factors include:

- Anterior versus posterior location
- Extent of pathology
- Involvement of basal cistern and middle cerebral vasculature
- Involvement of cranial nerves
- Dominant versus nondominant hemisphere

- Findings of cortical mapping in dominant hemisphere cases
- Location of dominant venous drainage: Labbe and sylvian veins
- Other lobar involvement, frontal, insular, occipital, intraventricular, cingulate
- Distortions created by the pathology that will retract normal brain.

Once these factors are considered, if all other factors are equal, the trajectory that uses natural fissures and openings, allows for the shortest dissection pathway through noneloquent brain, and allows the longest trajectory within the pathology is usually the best choice.

Further consideration should be given to preservation of optic radiations, and projections of the mesial temporal lobe. If the pathology does not compromise the hippocampus, the amygdala, or the afferent and efferent connections of these structures, care should be taken to preserve them. If, however, these structures and their connections are already irreversibly compromised, preservation of disconnected structures will not likely benefit the patient. For instance, a preserved hippocampus that is fully disconnected from the entorhinal cortex and the uncinate fasciculus is not likely to have useful function. Followed over time, the hippocampus will become atrophied, and may even contribute to seizures. Similarly, the major nuclei of the amygdala, the lateral, basal and accessory basal nuclei have their major inputs from the hippocampus. Thus, preserving of the amygdala with an absent hippocampus is not likely beneficial. The exception to this is the centromedian group that has major projections to the claustrum.

The major argument for preserving the amygdala in mesial temporal surgery is that the superior medial aspect of the amygdala and the semilunar gyrus of the uncus are immediately adjacent to the anterior choroidal artery usually found in the endorhinal sulcus, and the optic tract. However, careful use of these readily identifiable landmarks will allow for an aggressive resection of pathology in this area.

Further discussion of the surgical approaches and navigation of complex anatomy present in this area is presented in the case illustrations.

CASE 1: RIGHT-SIDED AMYGDALA AND HIPPOCAMPUS LOW GRADE GLIOMA

History

A 44-year-old right-handed male with history of generalized tonic clonic seizures arising from the right mesial temporal lobe. Preoperative evaluation did not reveal any abnormal spiking on electroencephalography of the lateral neocortical region.

Magnetic resonance imaging (MRI) (Figs. 3.9A to F) of the brain revealed a nonenhancing lesion involving the right anterior mesial temporal lobe in the uncus and hippocampal head. Superiorly, the tumor was noted to encroach the basal ganglia anteriorly. No enhancement was noted.

Thus, given the focal nature of the lesion, a selective amygdalohippocampectomy using a middle temporal gyrus approach was chosen.

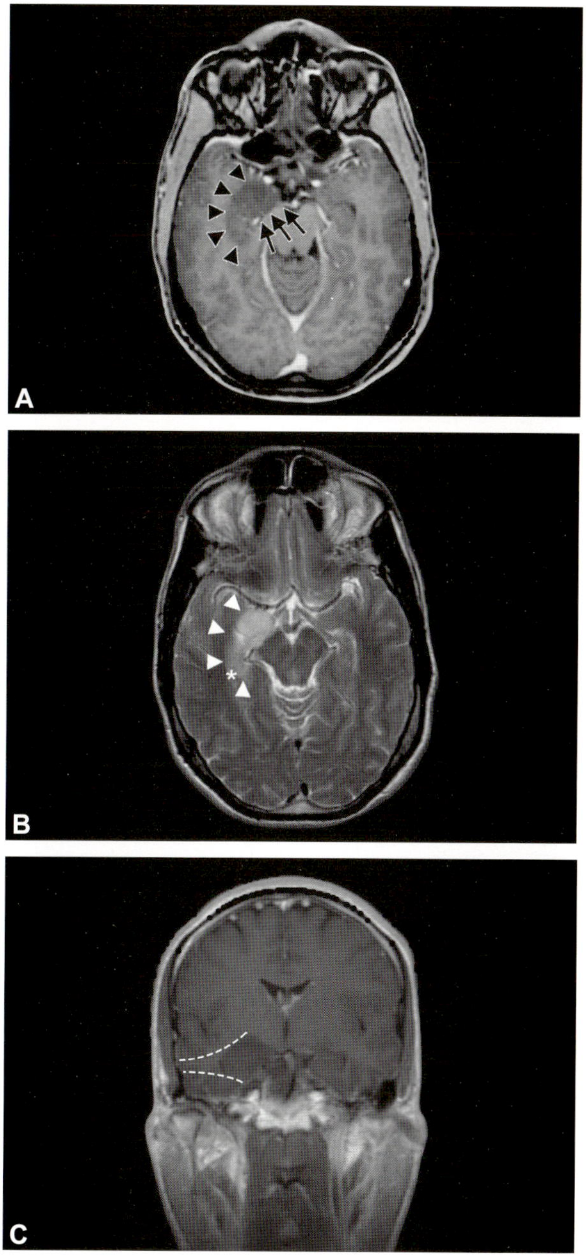

Figs. 3.9A to C: MRI of brain including T1 postcontrast and T2 preoperative (A to C) and postoperative (D to F) axial and coronal sections of the brain demonstrating nonenhancing lesion involving the right uncus and hippocampal head. (A) Axial T1 contrast enhanced sequence. The lesion appears medial to the temporal horn (arrowheads). Note the medial relationship to the posterior cerebral artery (PCA) and cerebral peduncle (arrows). (B) T2 axial section demonstrating a well-demarcated lesion with minimal edema. Arrowheads demonstrate the lateral margin of the tumor. Note the posteriorly displaced temporal horn (*). (C) Coronal postcontrast image showing the superior margin of the tumor. Dotted lines mark the keyhole middle temporal gyrus approach to the tumor.

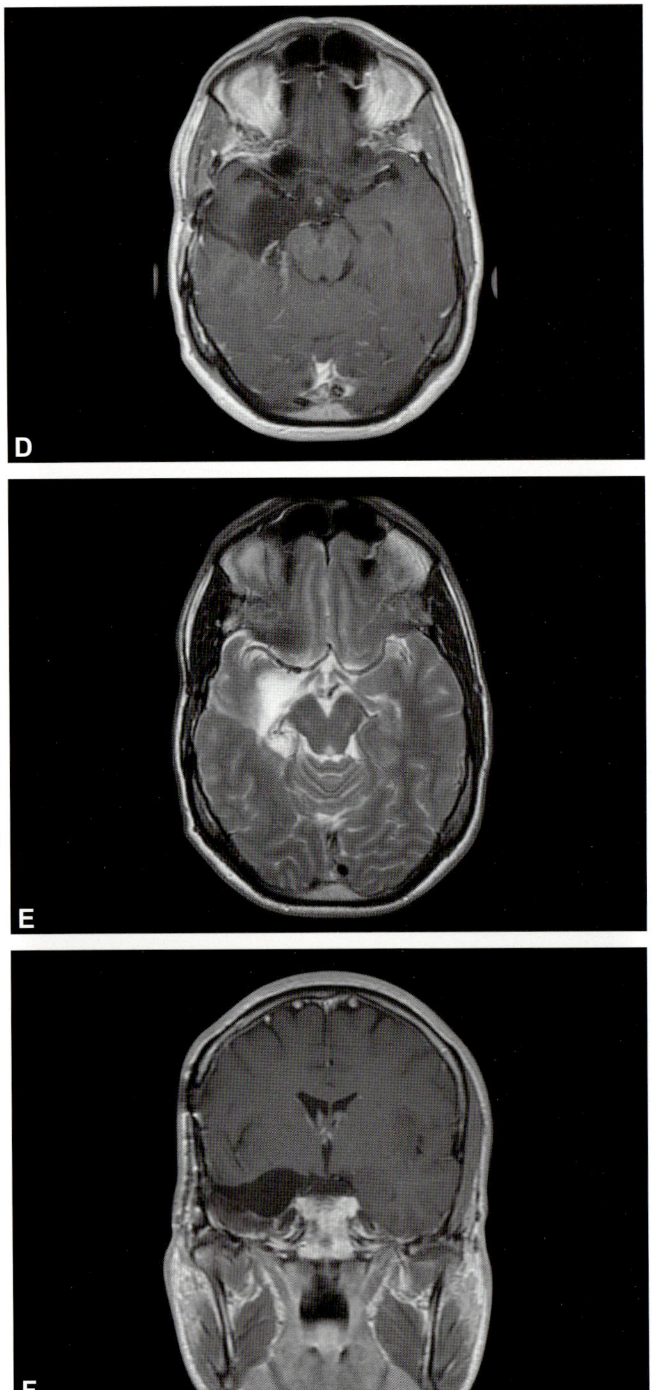

Figs. 3.9D to F: Corresponding postoperative sections obtained 6 months after surgery showing the resection cavity.

Surgery

After dural opening, a corticotomy was made along the middle temporal gyrus and dissection was carried down in the white matter until the collateral sulcus was identified. Dissection continued superiorly and medially until the ventricle was encountered. Tumor was readily visible (Figs. 3.10A to E).

Anteriorly, the rhinal sulcus was identified and the contents of the uncus were removed subpially. Posteriorly, the choroidal point was identified and the superior margin of tumor resection was identified using vascular landmarks by following the course of the anterior choroidal artery as the superior margin of resection. The tumor-laden hippocampal head and body were removed anatomically in two steps as previously described.

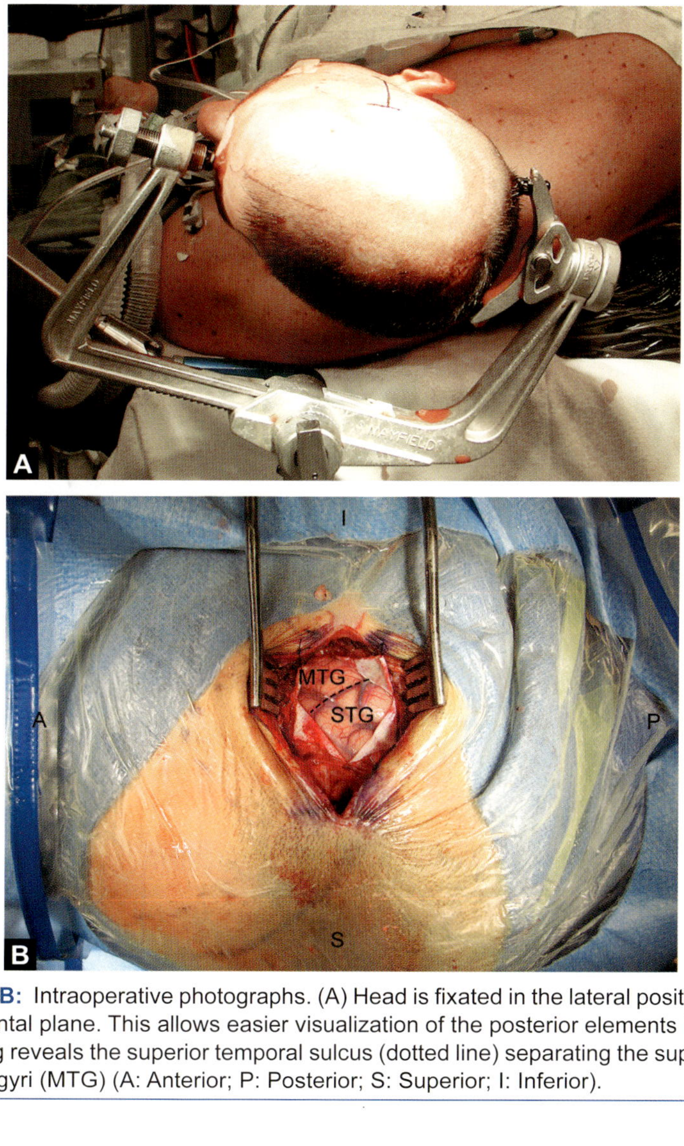

Figs. 3.10A and B: Intraoperative photographs. (A) Head is fixated in the lateral position with the nose 15° above the horizontal plane. This allows easier visualization of the posterior elements in the temporal horn. (B) Dural opening reveals the superior temporal sulcus (dotted line) separating the superior (STG) from the middle temporal gyri (MTG) (A: Anterior; P: Posterior; S: Superior; I: Inferior).

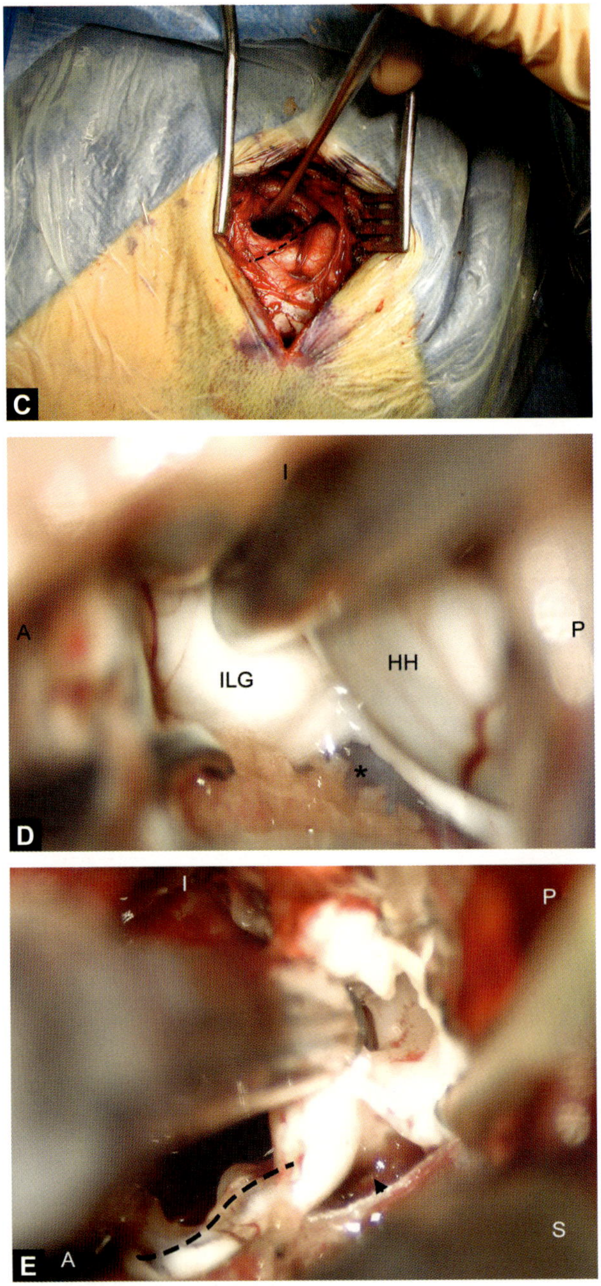

Figs. 3.10C to E: (C) A cortical approach through the middle temporal gyrus has been made. (D) Microscopic visualization of the intraventricular anatomy, allowing for anatomical resection of the lesion. The choroidal point (*) is readily identifiable after retraction of the choroid plexus. Immediately anterior to it is the intralimbic gyrus (ILG) which looks enlarged from the tumor. The hippocampal head (HH) is seen posteroinferiorly. (E) The anterior resection has been completed and the microscope is oriented posteriorly. The ultrasonic aspirator is removing the body of the hippocampus. The hippocampal sulcus remnant (dotted line) is visible. Note the posterior cerebral artery (PCA) perforators (arrowhead) visible through the pia. (A: Anterior; P: Posterior; S: Superior; I: Inferior)

CASE 2: LEFT UNCUS CAVERNOUS MALFORMATION

History

A 51-year-old right-handed male with history of generalized refractory epilepsy arising from the left temporal lobe who was found to have a cavernous malformation involving the uncus.

Magnetic resonance imaging (MRI) (Figs. 3.11A to D) of the brain revealed a lesion involving the anteromedial uncus abutting the sylvian fissure.

Thus, given the focal nature of the lesion and its proximity to the natural arachnoid plane of the sylvian fissure, a transsylvian approach to resection was planned.

Surgery

After dural opening, the sylvian fissure is identified and opened in subarachnoid plane. Given the anterior location of the cavernoma, an extensive opening of the fissure is not warranted.

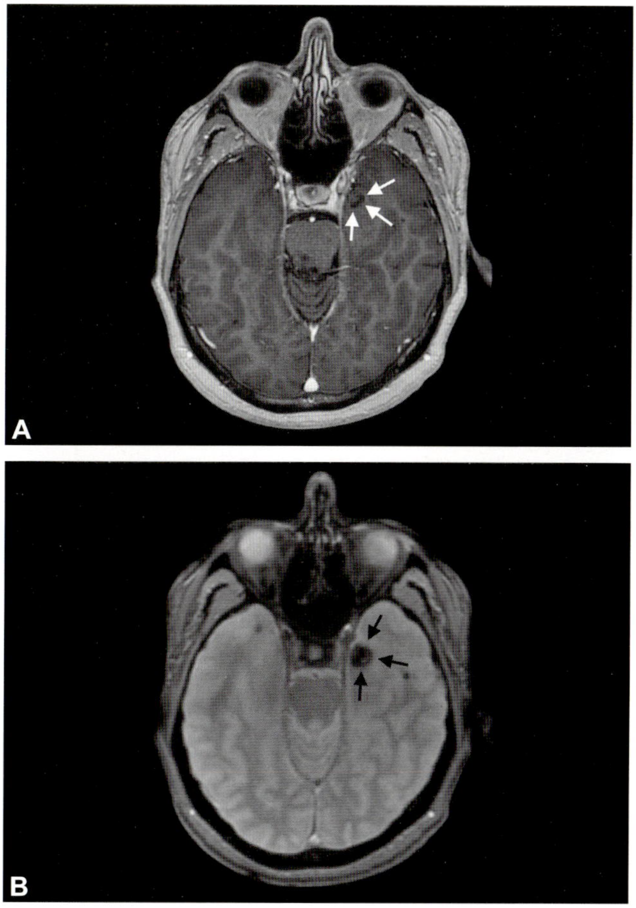

Figs. 3.11A and B: MRI studies. Preoperative T1 postcontrast (A) and Gradient Echo (B) sequences demonstrating the left anterior uncal lesion (arrows). Not the medial proximity to the Sylvian fissure and carotid artery.

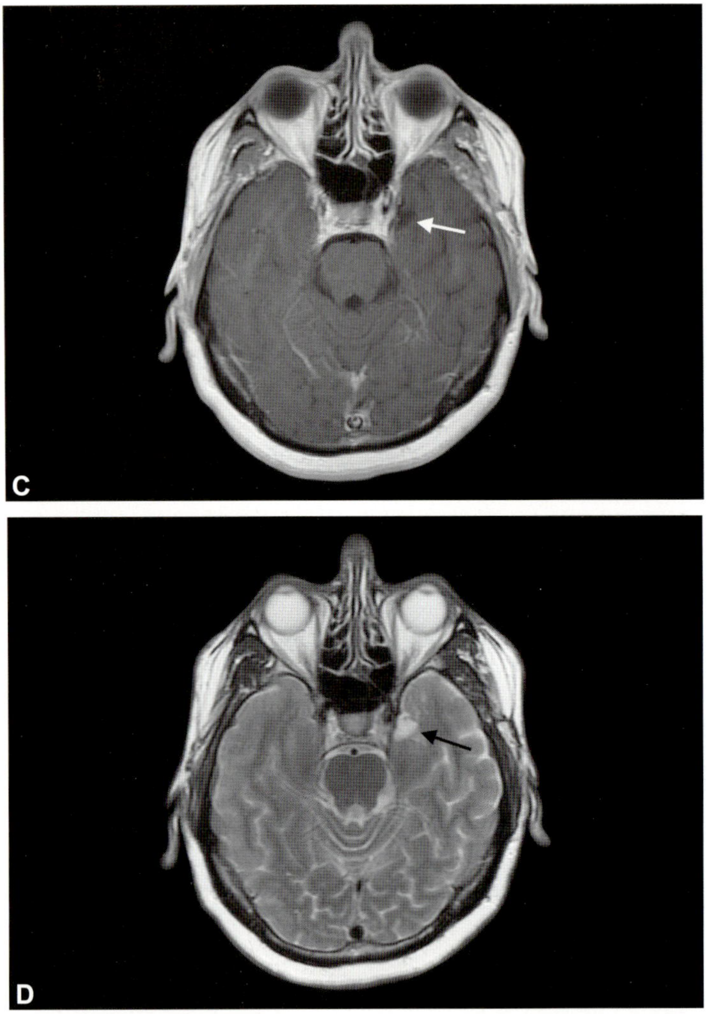

Figs. 3.11C and D: Postoperative T1 (C) and T2 (D) sequences demonstrate complete resection with no residual mass effect or edema. Note the resection cavity (arrow).

Rather, the triangular cistern is identified and fissure is opened anteriorly (Figs. 3.12A to D). Once the middle cerebral artery (MCA) bifurcation is identified, it is followed proximally until the internal carotid artery (ICA) is visualized and all arachnoid fibers are dissected. Attention is turned lateral where the uncal gyrus is readily visible. A corridor anterior to the anterior temporal artery is identified and corticotomy performed. Care is taken to avoid inadvertent injury to the Sylvia vein or branches.

Once the uncus is entered, dissection is carried laterally until the lesion is identified. Circumferential dissection, if possible, is preferred. Once removed, the uncal gyrus is emptied subpially to optimize a favorable seizure outcome.

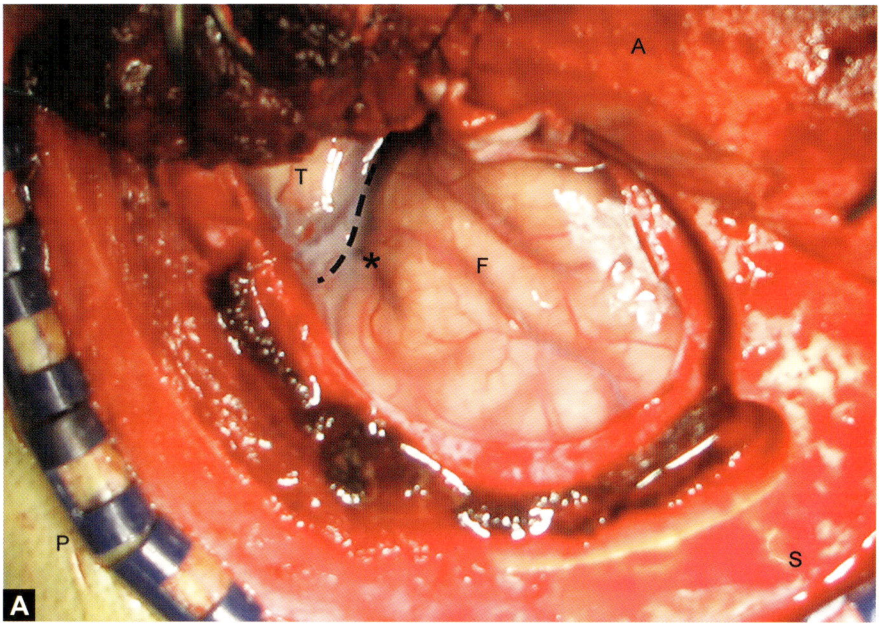

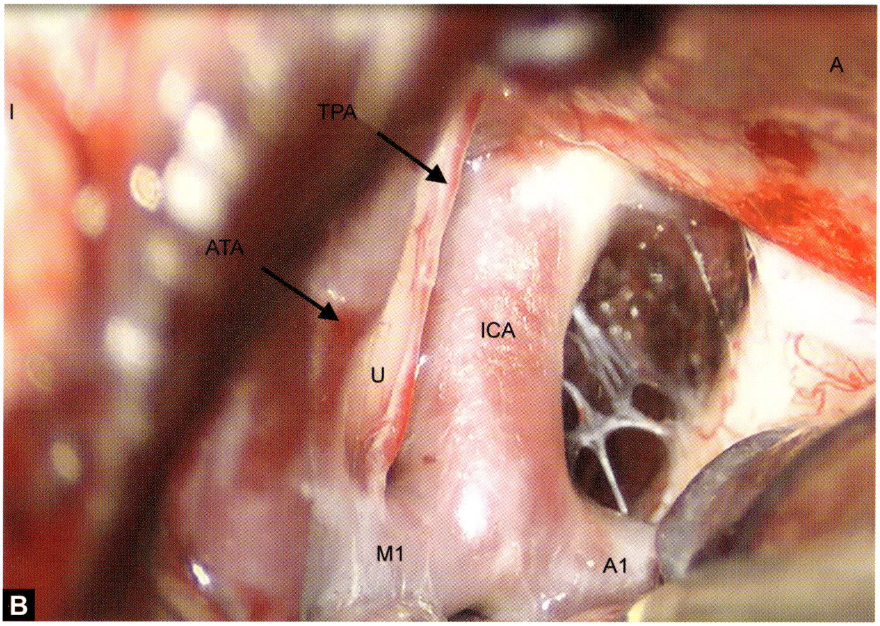

Figs. 3.12A and B: Intraoperative photographs. (A) Dura is opened and relevant anatomy identified (dotted line: Sylvian fissure; A: Anterior; P: Posterior; S: Superior; F: Frontal lobe; T: Temporal lobe; *: Triangular cistern of frontal operculum). (B) Sylvian fissure is dissected and attention is turned lateral to the internal carotid artery (ICA), before bifurcation to the middle cerebral (M1) and anterior cerebral (A1) arteries. The section of the uncus (U) between temporal polar artery (TPA) and anterior temporal artery (ATA) is visible. The operative window of uncal opening will be between these two arteries.

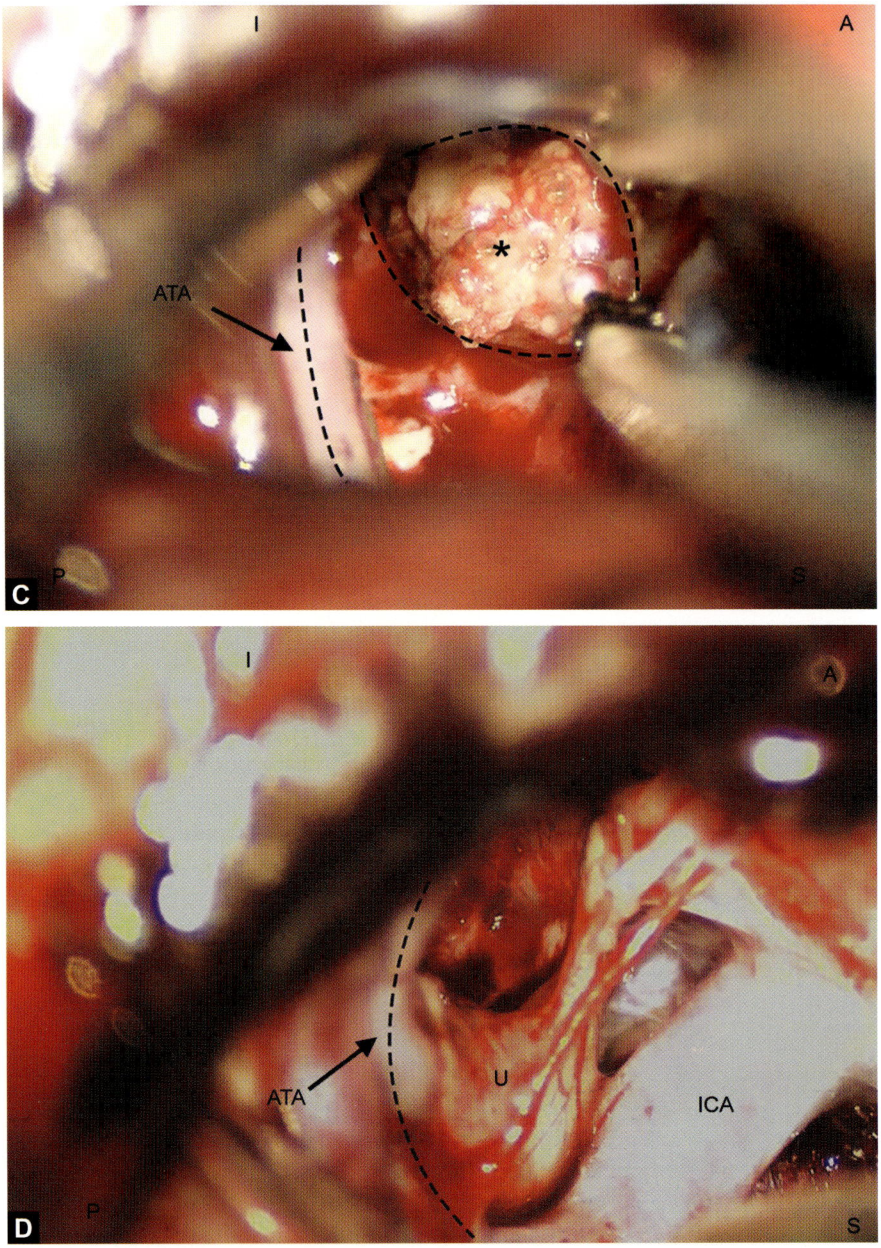

Figs. 3.12C and D: (C) Upon entering the uncus, dissection is carried until the lesion is identified. It is circumferentially dissected (*) before removal. (D) The cavity is visible within the surrounding anatomy. (ATA: Anterior temporal artery; U: Uncus; ICA: Internal cerebral artery; I: Inferior; A: Anterior; P: Posterior; S: Superior).

VIDEO LEGENDS

Videos 3.1 and 3.2: Microscopic resection of the mesial temporal lobe structures.

CHAPTER

4 Supracerebellar Transtentorial Approach to Limbic Tumors

Demi Dawkins, Ilhan Aydin, Kyle Swanson, Mustafa K Baskaya

HISTORY

Voight and Yasargil first described the supracerebellar transtentorial (SCTT) approach in 1976 as an alternative route to the posterior mediobasal temporal region containing the parahippocampal, fusiform, and lingula gyri as well as the isthmus of the cingulate gyrus.[1] It is a modification of the infratentorial approach first described by Oppenheimer and Krause.[2] Access to this region is quite difficult due to its deep location, important associated neurological pathways, and complex vascular anatomy. This approach was devised to reduce neurological deficits due to retraction or traversing cortical structures.[3] Yonekawa first described their series of this approach and demonstrated its ability to safely resect various lesions of this region.[4] This alternative approach has continued to be an excellent and safe corridor to access the posterior mediobasal temporal region. This chapter aims to outline this approach and emphasize its importance to the armamentarium of any neurosurgeon.

ANATOMY

Gross Anatomy

The SCTT approach is widely recognized for its ability to access lesions of the posterior mediobasal temporal region, which is part of the limbic system. It is composed of two main parts: (1) the paralimbic and (2) limbic areas. The paralimbic area consists of the temporal pole and parahippocampal gyrus. The limbic area consists of the amygdala, piriform cortex and retrocommissural portion of the hippocampal formation.[5] The cavernous sinus and carotid, crural, and ambient cisterns limit it medially. The lesser wing of the sphenoid bone and the isthmus of the cingulate gyrus and tip of the cuneus are the anterior and posterior limits, respectively. The lateral limit is the rhinal and collateral sulci.[5]

Most authors divide this region into three portions: (1) anterior, (2) middle, and (3) posterior.[6-8] There are some mild variations in the identified borders, but generally the imaginary line traversing the posterior limit of the uncus limits the anterior portion posteriorly, and the middle and posterior portions are separated by the quadrageminal plate.[5,7,9] The SCTT approach allows access to the posterior parahippocampal gyrus and the adjacent fusiform (occipitotemporal) gyrus, which are separated by the collateral sulcus. The anterior lingual gyrus of the occipital lobe can also be accessed. Finally, a transcollateral sulcus approach through SCTT can provide access to the atrium of the lateral ventricle, which is on average 1.3 cm deep to the collateral sulcus.[10]

There are important temporal and occipital structures that overly the mediobasal temporal region and can present potential obstacles in surgery if not properly recognized. The fronto-occipital fasciculus connects the frontal and occipital lobes and this tract can be identified with proper preoperative MRI sequencing. The optic radiations connect the lateral geniculate body to the occipital cortex and can be injured by direct transcortical approaches to the region or by retraction during subtemporal approaches.[5]

Vascular Anatomy

The middle and posterior cerebral arteries provide vascular supply to the mediobasal temporal region. The terminal posterior cerebral artery branches, parieto-occipital artery, and calcarine artery supply the posterior division.[7,9]

Venous drainage is achieved mainly via the basal vein of Rosenthal, which subsequently drains into the vein of Galen.[7,9] The basal vein of Rosenthal is located in the ambient cistern. Posteriorly, there is venous drainage into the torcula.[7]

Tentorium

The tentorium blankets the cerebellum and is fixed to the cranium except for the edges along the incisura. The anterior border attaches to the petrous ridge and encloses the superior petrosal sinus. The lateral and posterior borders attach to the occipital and temporal bones and encompass the transverse sinus and torcula. The attachment of the tentorium to the petrous apex and clinoid process forms three dural folds and between these folds lays the oculomotor trigone over the roof of the cavernous sinus. This is where the oculomotor and trochlear nerves enter the cavernous sinus. The tentorial incisura is triangular shaped. It is limited anteriorly by the dorsum sella and lies just posterior to the midbrain and pineal gland. Its contents include the midbrain, uncus, and parahippocampal gyrus.[11]

INDICATIONS

The SCTT approach can be utilized to tackle a wide variety of lesions including tumors, vascular malformations, posterior mesial temporal epilepsy, and can also provide a route to targets for vascular bypass. It provides a corridor to treat lesions of the posterior aspect of the medial basal temporal lobe (Figs. 4.1A to F), pineal region, upper brainstem, and can reach the atrium of the lateral ventricle.[5,10,12]

In cases of dominant hemisphere lesions, this approach offers a good alternative to subtemporal, transcortical, and interhemispheric approaches that may place eloquent speech and visual cortex at risk (Figs. 4.2A to D).[5,7,9,10] Specifically, the subtemporal and posterior occipital interhemispheric approaches require significant retraction on the temporal and occipital lobes, respectively.[5,7,9] The SCTT approach also preserves the optic radiations, which

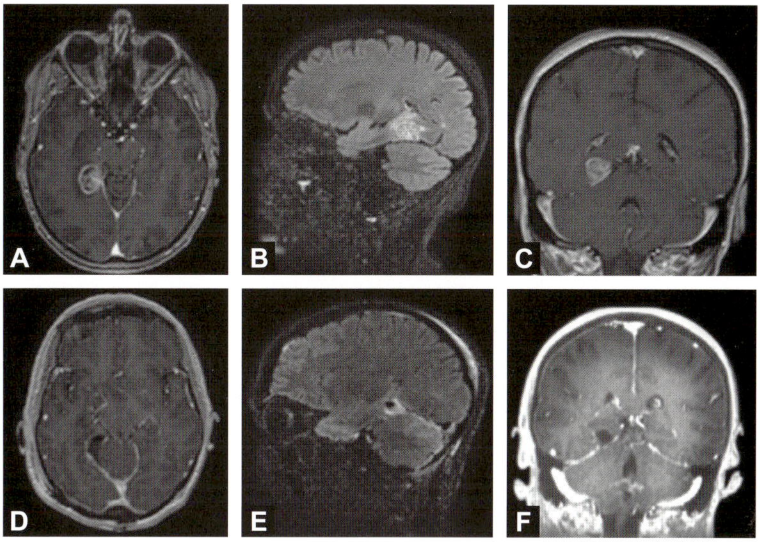

Figs. 4.1A to F: Magnetic resonance imaging (MRI) of a 53-year-old female presenting with seizures. Preoperative (A) axial T1 postcontrast, (B) sagittal T2 flair-cube, (C) coronal T1 postcontrast MRIs show a right-sided contrast enhancing mass lesion in the posterior parahippocampal region. Note relationship of the mass with the tentorium. Postoperative (D) axial T1 postcontrast, (E) sagittal T2 flair-cube, (F) coronal T1 postcontrast MRIs show gross total resection of grade IV astrocytoma after a supracerebellar transtentorial approach has been utilized.

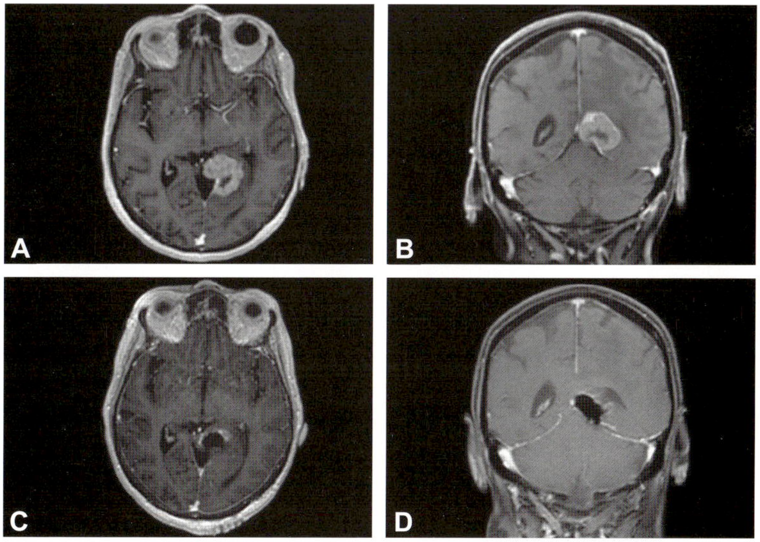

Figs. 4.2A to D: Magnetic resonance imaging (MRI) of a 71-year-old female with known lung cancer presenting with recent onset cognitive deficits. Preoperative (A) axial T1 postcontrast and (B) coronal T1 postcontrast MRIs show large left-sided contrast enhancing mass in the posterior parahippocampal region with extension towards to isthmus and cingulate gyrus. Postoperative (C) axial T1 postcontrast and (D) coronal T1 postcontrast MRIs show gross total resection of grade IV astrocytoma after a supracerebellar transtentorial approach has been utilized.

would be placed at risk during transcortical approaches.[5,9,10] Subtemporal and transtemporal approaches also pose risk of injury to the vein of Labbe.[7,9]

CONTRAINDICATIONS

Contraindications to this approach are based heavily on the surrounding anatomy. It may not provide a good access to the anterior division of the mediobasal temporal region unless a very large tumor extending from the posterior region has already made a space.[5-7] The inferior surface of the anterior parahippocampal gyrus is hidden by the petrous ridge, thus limiting this approach.[5,6] This can be circumvented by the use of curved endoscopes, but will significantly increase the degree of difficulty of this approach.[5,6] Large lesions with significant lateral, superior, or anterior extension may not be amenable to complete resection due to an inability to reach or visualize the entire lesion. For vascular pathology, in particular aneurysm or arteriovenous malformations (AVM), this approach can present some difficulty. For aneurysm surgery it is hard to obtain proximal arterial control and for AVM, early exposure of the venous drainage can be challenging due to the greater working distance and limitations in angles.[7] However, cavernous malformations located in the posterior mediobasal temporal region can be accessed via SCTT approach.[13] A steep tentorial angle can also be a relative contraindication to this approach. Careful attention should be paid to preoperative imaging.[6] If the basal vein of Rosenthal drains into the tentorium that would be a contraindication to the approach due to the significant risk of venous infarction during the tentorial incision.

DESCRIPTION OF THE APPROACH

Preoperative Evaluation and Positioning

There are two main positions for this approach—(1) sitting and (2) prone. The prone position is often preferred unless the body habitus make head flexion difficult because the preoperative evaluation for sitting can be more exhaustive than for the typical craniotomy. Consideration should be given for a transthoracic echocardiogram to evaluate for right to left shunting due to the risk of air embolism if utilizing the sitting position.[5,7] Intraoperatively, a transesophageal echogram probe or precordial Doppler can be placed to monitor for air embolism throughout the case at the discretion of the anesthesia team. At that time, an additional bubble test with Valsalva maneuver can be performed to evaluate for any shunting missed by the preoperative transthoracic echocardiogram.[5] Consider placing a central venous catheter at the beginning of the case so that any air may be aspirated if necessary.[9]

The most preferred and commonly described patient position is the sitting position with the head flexed with the goal of keeping the tentorium parallel to the floor.[6-8,13] There are many advantages to this position as gravity aids in the flow of cerebral spinal fluid (CSF), blood and irrigation out of the wound providing a clear operative field.[14] The sitting position also naturally permits less cerebellar retraction, as it will relax away with gravity. This position can be uncomfortable for the operating surgeon.[8] The semi-sitting position is an alternative that decreases the amount of back tilting and overall reduces the risk of air embolism.[5] The prone position may also be utilized in select patient populations, but at the expense of more cerebellar retraction. In this position the head is flexed, tilted away from the surgeon to maintain the natural anatomy and positioned higher than the level of the heart. It minimizes risk of air embolism and is more comfortable for the surgeon but can be difficult for the assistant surgeon.[3] We prefer the sitting position in obese patients or patients with a short neck which would preclude flexion and the prone position in patients with normal body habitus.

Placement of pins can vary with surgeon preference, but a good starting point would be placement of one pin on the mastoid of the contralateral side with two pins on the ipsilateral frontal and parietal regions.[5] On preoperative imaging, attention should be paid to the steepness of the tentorial angle, as this will affect positioning, degree of difficulty of the exposure, and surgeon comfort during dissection.[6,12] While obtaining the proper angle of the tentorium to the floor is important, the degree of neck flexion should not be so extreme as to compromise jugular venous outflow.[8] In the elderly population, care must be taken with neck manipulation as well.[5]

Incision and Craniotomy

The skin incision can either be vertical paramedian or a hockey-stick extension of a midline incision depending on surgeon preference and the target lesion. Although the leading author (Mustafa K Başkaya) initially used vertical median or paramedian incision, currently the hockey-stick extension provides wider exposure and results in less atrophy of muscles. For a midline approach, the incision should extend from the inion to the first or second cervical vertebra.[10] The paramedian incision passes through the midpoint of the imaginary line connecting the external occipital protuberance to the mastoid process.[14] The paramedian incision may be preferred for more laterally located lesions and reduces risk of injury to important midline venous structures.[4,12,15] In a paramedian approach, the bellies of the fronto-occipital and suboccipital muscles are split. Care should be taken to coagulate the occipital artery, which can be found in the layer beneath splenius capitis.[5] The hockey-stick extension of a midline incision allows subperiosteal dissection of muscles in the midline and allows for a craniotomy that is centered more to the side of the lesion (Figs. 4.3A and B), although in some cases with small lesions we use straight vertical incision as well.[10]

The craniotomy should be wide enough for exposure of the transverse sinus and torcula to prevent the bone overhang from limiting the degree of sinus retraction. The location of the transverse sinus can be predicted by the inion and superior nuchal line (Fig. 4.4).[11] With the availability of intraoperative neuronavigation these venous structures can be mapped out for proper placement of the burr holes and subsequent craniotomy. Two burr holes should be placed just superior to the transverse sinus and torcula and inferiorly two burr holes over the superior aspect of the cerebellum. The craniotomy can be extended to the transverse sigmoid junction laterally, but often this wide of an exposure is not needed.[7,9] The craniotomy should extend one-third above the transverse sinus and two-thirds below as well as two-thirds lateral to the torcula and one-third across midline (Fig. 4.5).[7,10] Care should be taken laterally to avoid exposure of the mastoid air cells. Regardless of whether or not these cells are truly opened, bone wax should be applied to the craniotomy edges to prevent CSF leak and decrease the risk of air embolism.[5]

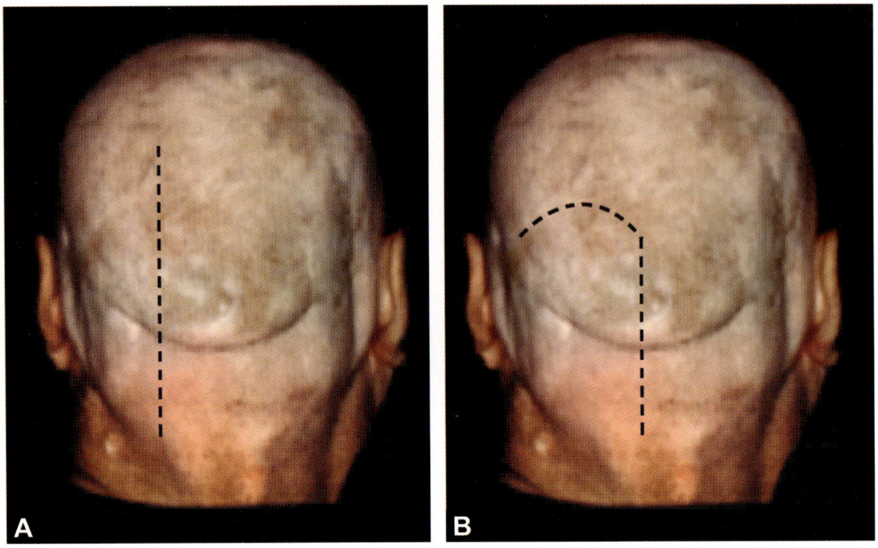

Figs. 4.3A and B: Preferred skin incisions are demonstrated in cadaveric heads. (A) A paramedian incision just lateral to midline, eccentric to the side of the lesion, passes through the midpoint of the imaginary line connecting the external occipital protuberance (inion) to the mastoid process. (B) A hockey stick incision eccentric to the side of the lesion, allows for further expansion of the exposure.

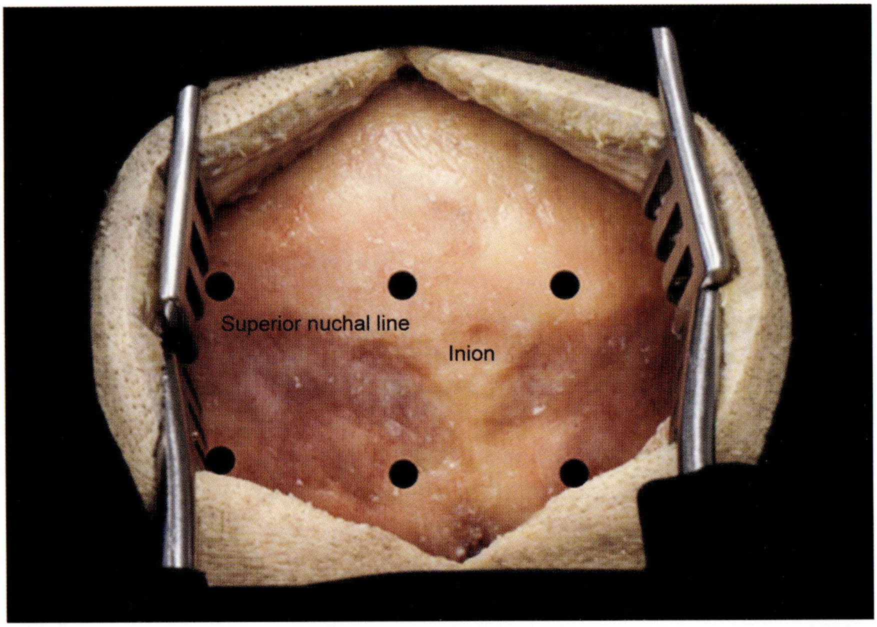

Fig. 4.4: Occipital bone exposure for craniotomy. The surface landmarks of the inion (external occipital protuberance) and the superior nuchal line can predict the location of the transverse sinus. Burr holes should be located just superior to the transverse sinus and torcula as well as over the superior aspect of the cerebellum.

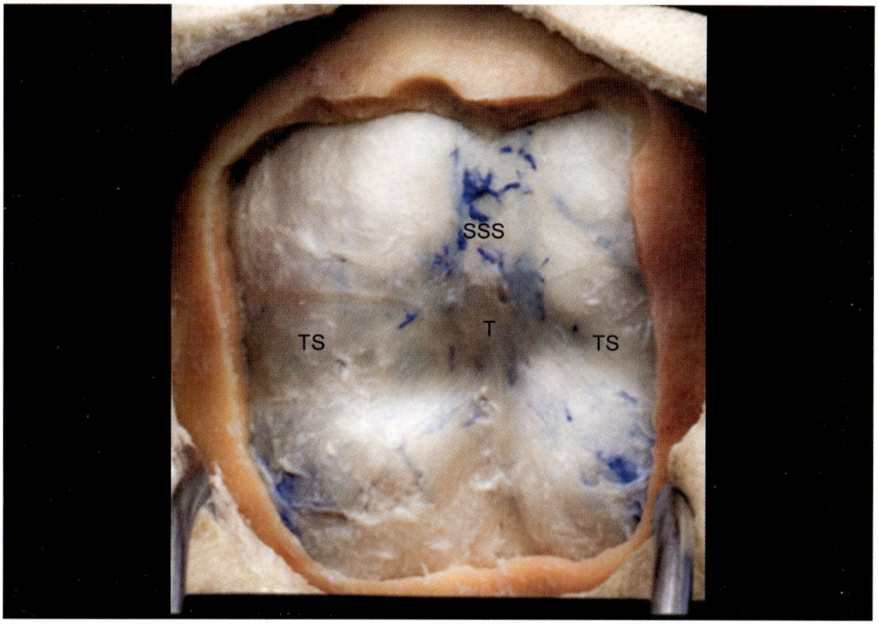

Fig. 4.5: Dural exposure following craniotomy. The opening exposes the dura one-third above the transverse sinus and two-thirds below.
(SSS: Superior sagittal sinus; T: Torcula; TS: Transverse sinus).

Dural Opening and Dissection

After completion of the desired craniotomy the dural opening may be achieved via a shallow U-shaped or V-shaped incision, with the dural opening extending to the transverse sinus and torcula (Figs. 4.6A and B).[12] This will allow the sinuses to be retracted superiorly with the dura and will significantly increase operative visualization.[10,13] The inferior aspect of the durotomy should only include the superior half of the dura overlying the occipital surface of the cerebellum in order to prevent outward cerebellar herniation.[7,10] The dura can be opened across the midline, with vascular clips or suture being used to control bleeding from the occipital sinus.[10] For the midline approach, some authors advocate reflecting the dura in two hemispheric flaps in order to preserve the occipital sinus,[14] though we feel this limits visualization. While performing the dural opening it is critical to not enter the transverse sinus. However, if this is done inadvertently, proper materials should be readily available to reduce risk of air embolism. CSF may be drained from the cisterna magna and dorsal mesencephalic cistern to relax the cerebellum.[5,7,14] If using the sitting position, gravity will assist with retraction of the cerebellum.[7] This cerebellar relaxation will open the corridor between the cerebellum and overlying tentorium. Additionally, releasing the adhesions of the arachnoid villi further opens this corridor.[13]

Bridging veins should be identified and can be sacrificed by coagulating near the cerebellar surface of the tentorium.[7,9] Preservation of the superior and inferior vermian veins located medially is essential to prevent venous infarct or hemorrhage, as these are the main veins draining the posterior fossa.[5,7] The use of the paramedian approach can be useful to avoid

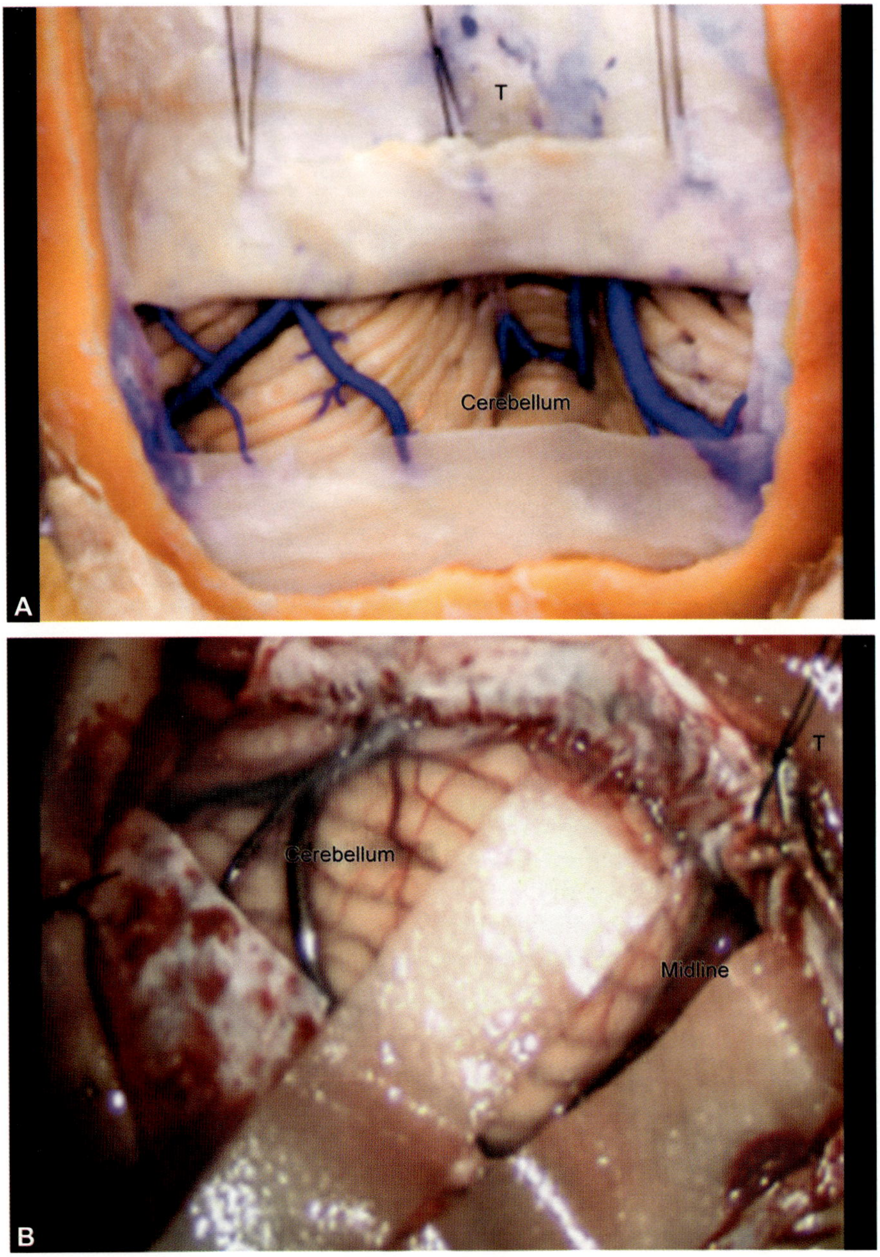

Figs. 4.6A and B: Dural opening (A) in the cadaveric dissection or (B) in real time case demonstrated here with a U-shaped incision. The transverse sinus is included superiorly and sutures applied provide retraction. Only the superior aspect of the suboccipital surface of the cerebellum is exposed to prevent outward herniation. This anatomical dissection demonstrates opening the occipital sinus to cross midline. (T: Torcula).

these midline structures.[5] If the borders of the transverse and petrosal sinus are followed, the trochlear nerve should be observed entering the free border of the tentorium.[9,11] Dissection

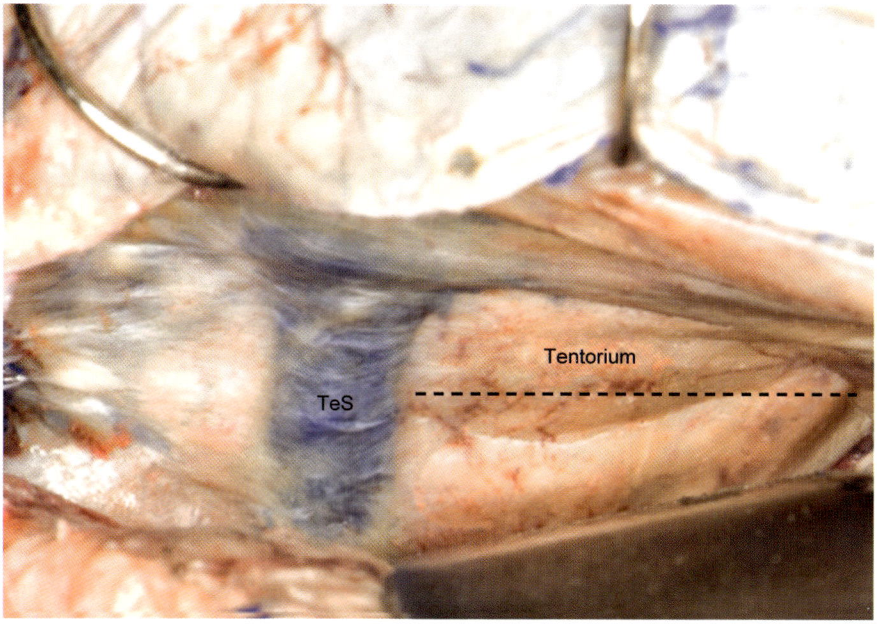

Fig. 4.7: Surgical corridor following retraction of the cerebellum inferiorly. The tentorial sinus is identified in the midline and should be preserved. A wide tentorial opening is outlined lateral to midline. (TeS: Tentorial sinus).

will be carried out to open the posterior aspect of the quadrageminal and ambient cisterns and the superior cerebellar artery and trochlear nerve should be identified. The trochlear nerve will be located laterally between the superior cerebellar artery and posterior cerebral artery after emerging from the dorsal aspect of the crus cerebri.[5] The trochlear nerve will then enter the brainstem inferior to the inferior colliculi.[7] Typically these structures do not need to be identified as intraoperative neuronavigation assists in locating the projection of the lesion on the tentorium. The tentorium is then opened lateral to the lesion.

Preoperatively attention should be paid to the venous anatomy within the tentorium to plan for the opening in the tentorium. The tentorium may contain a single large vein or multiple venous lakes and sinuses. Inadvertent opening of these may result in excessive blood loss. Precautions such as having vascular clips available should be taken before incising the tentorium. Moreover, rarely the vein of Labbé may drain into one of these tentorial sinuses. Therefore, preoperative knowledge on venous anatomy is of great importance (Figs. 4.7 and 4.8).[16] Good understanding of the trochlear nerve anatomy is also important to avoid inadvertent injury.[9] There have been reports of arrhythmias with the tentorial cut due to trigeminal nerve irritation so the anesthesia team should be warned at this point.[4,6] The tentorium should be incised 2–3 cm posterolateral from the posterior part of the tentorial incisura (Figs. 4.7 and 4.8).[5] The free edge of the tentorium can then be retracted with the superior cerebellar surface or resected (Figs. 4.9 and 4.10).[12] Arachnoid dissection in the quadrageminal cistern should be carried out taking care to preserve the branches of the posterior cerebral artery supplying the posterior division of the mediobasal temporal region.[10,12]

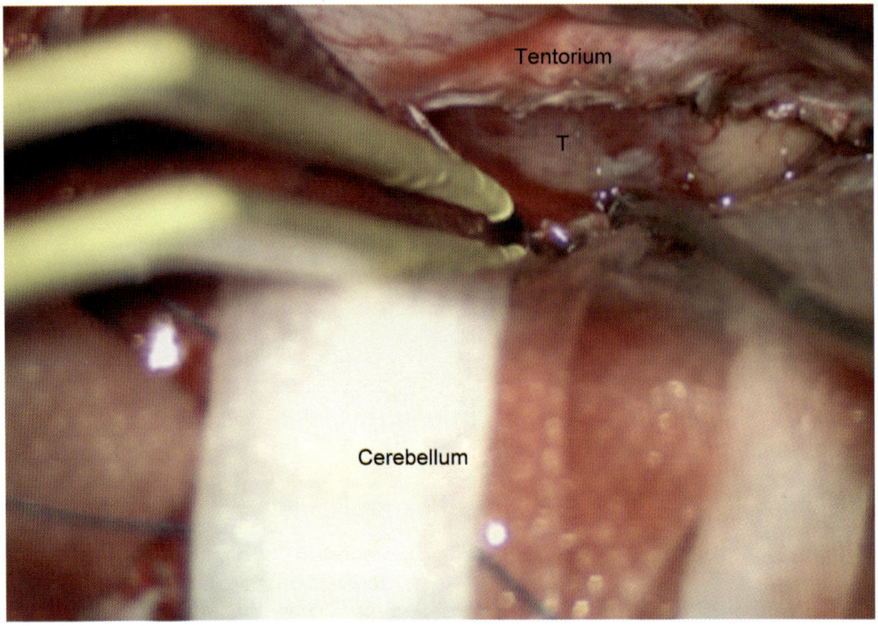

Fig. 4.8: After opening of the tentorium, the tumor in the posterior parahippocampal gyrus is exposed. Suction and bipolar forceps is retracting tentorial surface of the cerebellum.
(T: Tumor).

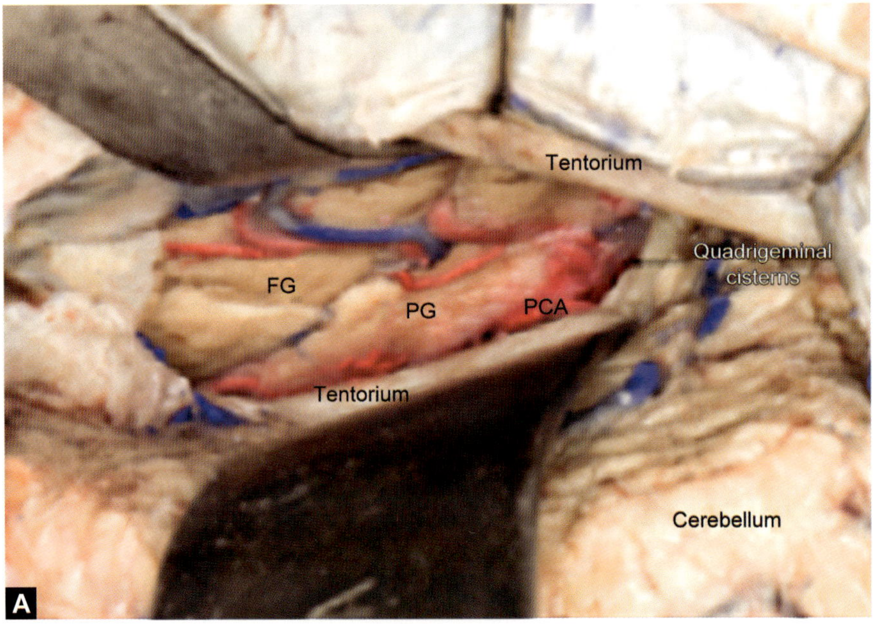

Fig. 4.9A

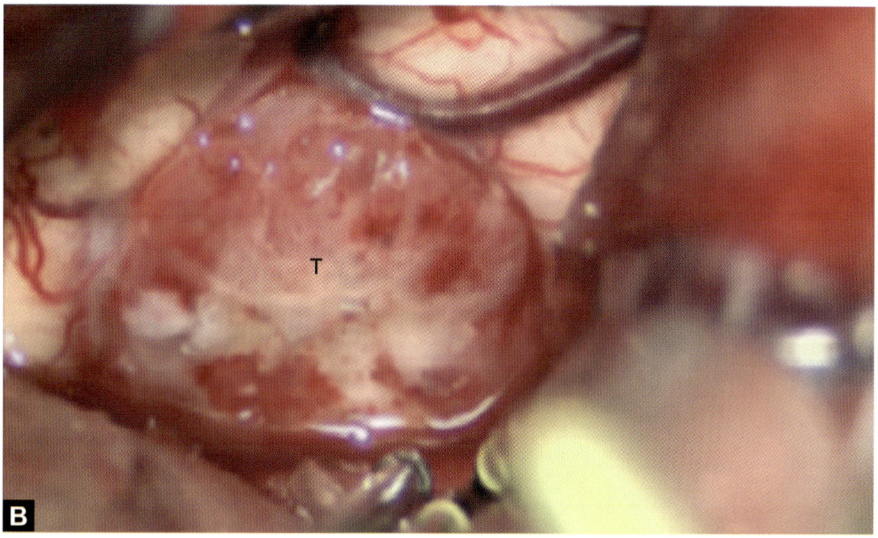

Figs. 4.9A and B: Surgical corridor following tentorial incision (A) in a cadaveric dissection and (B) in case with parahippocampal tumor. The tentorium is retracted inferiorly along with the cerebellum. This provides exposure of the posterior portion of the mediobasal temporal region including the fusiform and parahippocampal gyri. The posterior aspects of the ambient and quadrigeminal cisterns are exposed. The quadrigeminal segment of the posterior cerebral artery traverses at the inferior aspect of the field. Retraction on the tentorium increases the exposure. Note that no static retraction is applied on the cerebellum. (FG: Fusiform gyrus; PG: Parahippocampal gyrus; PCA: Posterior cerebral artery; T: Tumor).

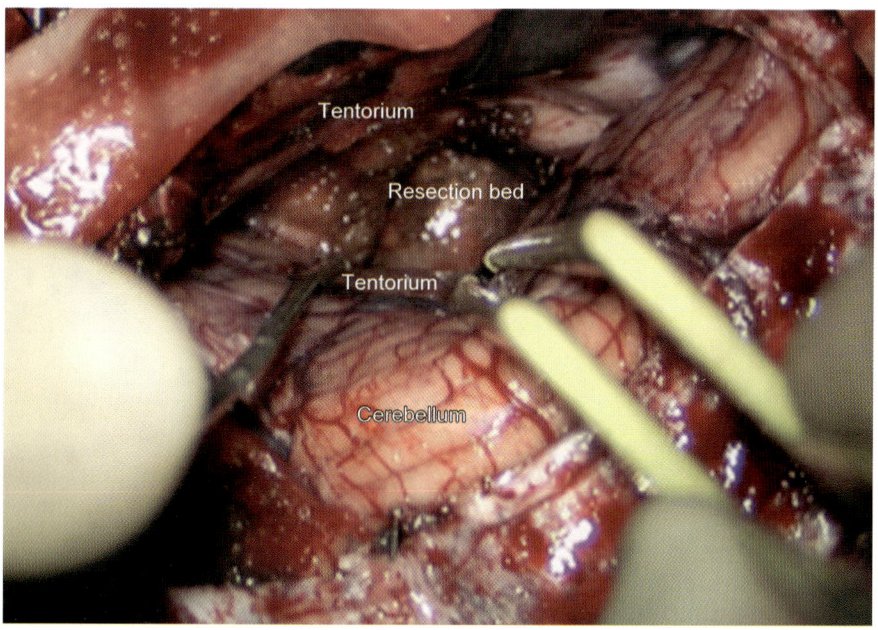

Fig. 4.10: Intraoperative photograph shows resection bed covered with a layer of surgicel after gross total resection of the tumor.

As an adjuvant to the traditional microscopic SCTT approach, endoscopic-assistance has been utilized for better visualization and more comfortable operating position. Specifically, the use of angled endoscopes allows for improved views around curves and corners that would typically limit this approach. It does require comfort with the use of endoscopy.[17] Figures 4.11A and B depict the intraoperative views gained by endoscopic assistance.

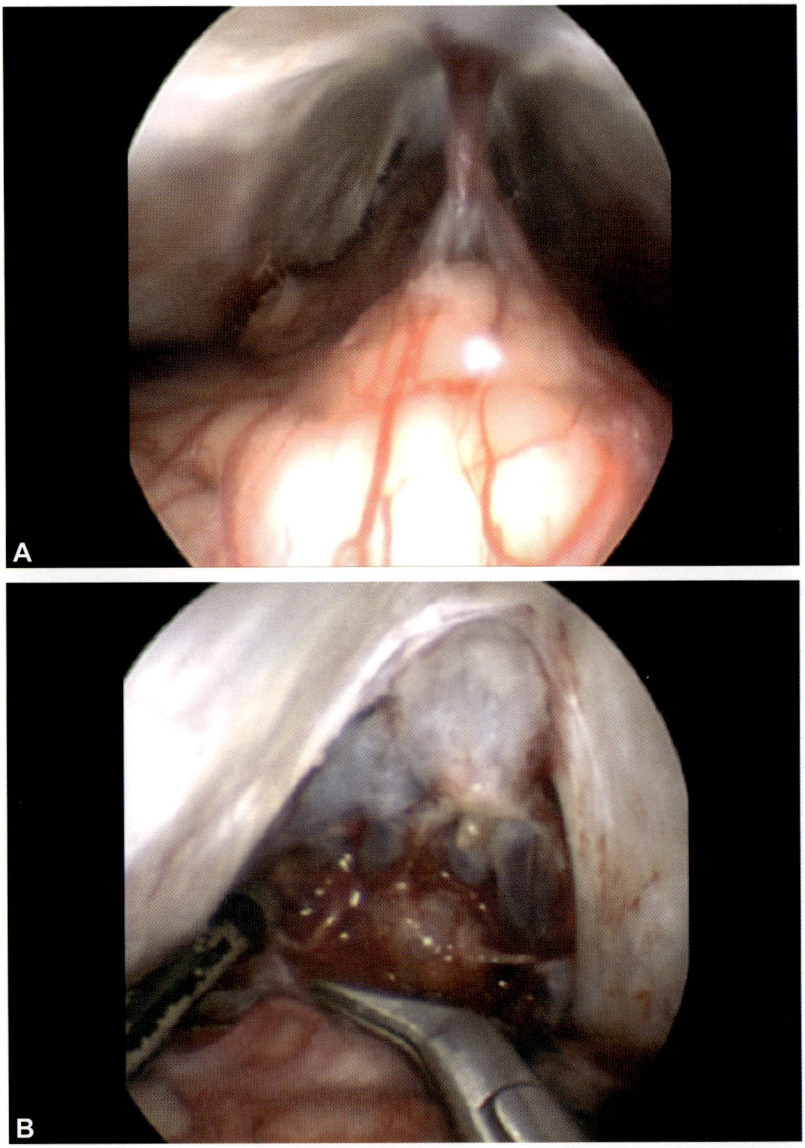

Figs. 4.11A and B: Endoscopic assistance allows for improved visualization. (A) Demonstrates a midline-bridging vein, which will be sacrificed. (B) Depicts the vein of Galen in the midline draining the basal vein of Rosenthal and internal cerebral veins. The pineal gland is located inferiorly.
Courtesy: Dr Azam Ahmed.

Closure

The free edge of the tentorium can be restored with either suture or glue as described by Yonekawa, but generally we have not found this necessary and prefer to leave the tentorium open.[4] Watertight dural closure is imperative to prevent development of a pseudomeningocele or CSF leak. Duroplasty can be performed with pericranium harvested during the opening or with a dural substitute.[10] We also utilize dural sealant to decrease the likelihood of CSF leak. The head of bed should be kept elevated postoperatively to improve wound healing.[5]

RISKS AND PITFALLS

One of the most concerning risks of this approach is air embolism due to violation of the sinuses while in the sitting position. This may be avoided, if performed in the prone position, but this position may not be ideal for all patient populations. Along with very vigilant preoperative evaluation, proper knowledge of identification of air embolism, along with the appropriate interventions is important. Early signs of air embolism include sudden decrease in end-tidal CO_2, oxygen desaturation, increase in blood pressure, ventricular dysrhythmia, or increase in central venous pressures.[5] It is important to have an experienced anesthesiology team while performing this approach.

As with any surgery intricate knowledge of the surrounding anatomy is critical. The landmarks in this region are fairly simple to identify, but it does require a familiarity with a different perspective of the approach to the posterior mediobasal temporal region.[5] The tentorial incision can be difficult both due to the venous and cranial nerve anatomy of this region. The venous anatomy of this region must be reviewed on preoperative imaging. Occasionally, a large venous sinus can be present within the tentorium and it can make this approach significantly more difficult.[9] Also venous drainage of the cerebellum relies heavily of the vermian veins so these should not be sacrificed to avoid venous infarct or hemorrhage.[5,9] Use of the paramedian approach can be helpful in preservation of this important venous structure.[5,12] A good understanding of the trochlear nerve anatomy is also important to avoid injury with resection of the tentorium. If the border of the transverse sinus and petrosal sinus are followed, the trochlear nerve will be identified entering the free border.[9]

For most lesions a median incision will be preferred to eliminate dissection of the suboccipital musculature.[9] If, however, a paramedian approach is necessary care should be taken to properly divide the muscle bellies to reduce muscle atrophy and neck pain.[5,7]

Main limitations of this approach are the lesions located in the middle third or anterior third of mediobasal temporal region and the lesion extending superiorly to the posterior portion of the cingulate gyrus through isthmus. Case example with these limitations is presented in a separate chapter (Giant Limbic Tumors).

REFERENCES

1. Voight K, Yaşargil M. Cerebral cavernous haemangiomas or cavernomas. Neurochirurgia (Stuttg). 1976;19(2):59-68.
2. Ziyal IM, Ozgen T. Transtentorial approach to posterior temporomedial structures. J Neurosurg. 2001;95(3):541.

3. Kobayashi S, Sugita K, Tanaka Y, Kyoshima K. Infratentorial Approach to the Pineal Region in the Prone Position: Concorde Position. J Neurosurg. 1983;58(1):141-3.
4. Yonekawa Y, Imhof HG, Taub E, Curcic M, Kaku Y, Roth P, et al. Supracerebellar transtentorial approach to posterior temporomedial structures. J Neurosurg. 2001;94(2):339-45.
5. Türe U, Harput MV, Kaya AH, Baimedi P, Firat Z, Türe H, et al. The paramedian supracerebellar-transtentorial approach to the entire length of the mediobasal temporal region: an anatomical and clinical study. J Neurosurg. 2012;116(4):773-91.
6. Lafazanos S, Türe U, Harput MV, Gonzalez Lopez P, Fırat Z, Türe H, et al. Evaluating the importance of the tentorial angle in the paramedian supracerebellar-transtentorial approach for selective amygdalohippocampectomy. World Neurosurg. 2015;83(5):836-41.
7. Moftakhar R, Izci Y, Başkaya MK. Microsurgical anatomy of the supracerebellar transtentorial approach to the posterior mediobasal temporal region. Neurosurgery. 2008;62(3 Suppl 1):1-7.
8. Suslu HT, Bozbuga M, Ozturk A, Sahinoglu K. Surface anatomy of the transverse sinus for the midline infratentorial supracerebellar approach. Turk Neurosurg. 2010;20(1):39-42.
9. de Oliveira JG, Párraga RG, Chaddad-Neto F, Ribas GC, de Oliveira EP. Supracerebellar transtentorial approach—resection of the tentorium instead of an opening—to provide broad exposure of the mediobasal temporal lobe: anatomical aspects and surgical applications. J Neurosurg. 2012;116(4):764-72.
10. Izci Y, Seçkin H, Ateş O, Başkaya MK. Supracerebellar transtentorial transcollateral sulcus approach to the atrium of the lateral ventricle: microsurgical anatomy and surgical technique in cadaveric dissections. Surg Neurol. 2009;72(5):509-14.
11. Rhoton AL. Tentorial incisura. Neurosurgery. 2000;47(3):S131-53.
12. Jittapiromsak P, Deshmukh P, Nakaji P, Spetzler RF, Preul MC. Comparative analysis of posterior approaches to the medial temporal region. Neurosurgery. 2009;64(3):ons35-42.
13. Swanson KI, Cikla U, Uluc K, Baskaya MK. Supracerebellar transtentorial approach to the tentorial incisura and beyond. Neurosurg Focus. 2016;40(Video Suppl)1:2016.
14. Yaşargil MG, Abernathey CD. Microneurosurgery. Stuttgart: Thieme; 1996.
15. Uchiyama N, Hasegawa M, Kita D, Yamashita J. Paramedian supracerebellar transtentorial approach for a medial tentorial meningioma with supratentorial extension: technical case report. Neurosurgery. 2001;49(6):1470-3.
16. Avci E, Dagtekin A, Akture E, Uluc K, Baskaya MK. Microsurgical anatomy of the vein of Labbe. Surg Radiol Anat. 2011;33(7):569-73.
17. Villanueva P, Louis RG, Cutler AR, Wei H, Sale D, Duong HT, et al. Endoscopic and gravity-assisted resection of medial temporo-occipital lesions through a supracerebellar transtentorial approach. Operative Neurosurg. 2015;11(4):475-83.

CHAPTER

5

Surgical Approaches to the Insula

Sepehr Sani, Richard W Byrne

INTRODUCTION

The term insula is Latin for "island". This may indicate that early anatomists considered the insula to be isolated anatomically and functionally. Although Broca's patient, Louis Victor Leborgne, had suffered a stroke in his posterior inferior frontal gyrus, the stroke also affected his anterior insula. This was not, however, considered to be a speech area at the time. As there were few examples of isolated insula lesions it was difficult for neuroscientists to identify specific functions of the insula. Seizures and auras emanating from the insula gave some clues to the gustatory connections of the insula. Over time, with experience in insular surgery and with metabolic imaging techniques, it has become clear that the insula is widely interconnected with wide areas of the brain, and has at least a supportive role in many brain functions. Because of this, temporary function loss after a large insular resection is common. Autonomic functions, neurobehavioral functions, speech connectivity and the wide connections of the claustrum are among the known functions of the insula.

Nonetheless, it has become clear through experience that resections of the insular cortex that spare the vasculature and the internal capsule are usually well-tolerated. This was not the case in the past, prior to the advent of microsurgery and modern imaging. As such, prior to the modern microsurgical era, insular surgery was appropriately uncommon due to valid concerns over the potential for morbidity. Using microsurgery, image guidance and intraoperative monitoring, specific pathology of the insula including cavernous malformations, small arteriovenous malformations (AVMs) and low- or high-grade gliomas can be safely removed.

SURGICAL ANATOMY OF THE INSULA

The keys to safe surgery in the insula are many. First, the anatomy is not commonly encountered by general neurosurgeons. In order to safely operate in the insula, a deep commitment to understanding the anatomy of the region is essential. Second, since most approaches to the insula require a very wide splitting of the sylvian fissure despite the presence of insular pathology and careful manipulation of the middle cerebral artery (MCA) and its many branches, a patient and experienced microsurgeon is required. Finally, a familiarity with the techniques of awake surgery, cortical and subcortical mapping, and a commitment to study of the position of the lenticulostriate arteries and the internal capsule in three dimensions is essential.

Insular Anatomy

The insula has an irregular shape that is roughly similar to an inverted obtuse triangle with its obtuse angle at its anterior inferior base. It bulges out laterally and follows the internal capsule as its deep border. The shape of the lateral borders is relatively straightforward, as it follows the circular sulcus inferiorly and superiorly. These borders separate the insula from the temporal stem inferiorly and the white matter of the centrum semiovale and the operculum superiorly. Anteriorly, the insula terminates as the accessory gyrus of the insula just below pars orbitalis. Posteriorly, it terminates at the junction between the superior and inferior circular sulci. The insula is buried beneath the operculum in the adult, but early in human development, it exists as a surface structure and its own lobe. Because of this, many call the insula the fifth cerebral lobe. Clues to the surface anatomy of the insula lie in the study of its development. Initially, the insula appears as a smooth surface. By week 18 an angled central sulcus appears at the midpoint of the insula, rising as it moves posteriorly. This sulcus parallels the central sulcus of the lateral hemisphere. The central artery of the insular central sulcus also parallels the early branch of the central artery of the central sulcus, arising from the superior branch of the MCA. Anterior to the central sulcus are the short insular gyri with the accessory insular gyrus most anteriorly. Each of the insular gyri projects toward the insular pole, just behind the limen insula. Posterior to the central insular sulcus are the two long insular gyri, both rising from anterior to posterior and terminating just anterior to Heschl's gyrus and the two buried transverse temporal gyri of the posterior superior temporal plane. When followed medially, this terminal angle of the insular sulcus leads to the atrium of the ventricle approximately 2 cm deep and posterior. The long terminal branches of the inferior MCA penetrate the long insular gyri to bring blood supply to the posterior limb of the internal capsule, therefore identifying these structures is crucial. Any resection of the posterior insula must preserve these penetrating branches.

The blood supply to the anterior insula arises from the superior branch of the MCA. The many opercular branches of the superior branch of the MCA must be carefully preserved. The small terminal branches to the insula in the anterior half of the insula can be sacrificed while removing an insular lesion since these small branches to the insular cortex do not go to the genu or the posterior limb of the internal capsule. It should be remembered, however, that the majority of the large branches of the superior MCA are bypassing the insula on their way to terminate in the operculum. This is especially easy to miss in the triangular cistern, where bypassing opercular branches run in the vertical and horizontal sulcal rami of the triangular cistern. After splitting the sylvian fissure widely from inferior to superior insular sulci, an early dissection of the superior branch of the MCA will show that unlike the inferior branch of the MCA, which runs closely parallel to the inferior insular sulcus, the superior branch does not reach the superior insular sulcus. The superior branch of the MCA approaches the superior insular sulcus and then doubles back out over the apex of the insula just below the triangular cistern.

Following the middle cerebral artery from origin to its entry into the sylvian fissure is a useful way to study the anterior-inferior surface anatomy of the insula since preserving the branches and perforators of the MCA is one of the keys to insular surgery. The proximal MCA gives off the lenticulostriate branches from its posterior superior surface starting at the carotid bifurcation and extending to within 1.5 cm of the limen insula. The limen insula is the anterior inferior aspect of the insula that marks the entry of the distal M1 branch into the sylvian fissure. In most patients the MCA bifurcates just distal to the limen insula and, with the two branches separated by the insular pole, just superior and posterior to limen insula. The superior branch of the MCA rises to the insular apex under the pars triangularis of the frontal operculum. The inferior branch of the MCA runs in the inferior circular sulcus, below the insular apex.

Naturally large tumors or vascular malformations in this area will distort the anatomy and displace the MCA branches. If the lesion is primarily of the temporal lobe and the temporal stem extending into the insula, the inferior MCA may be dramatically elevated. This may give a temporal transcortical approach some advantages over a transsylvian approach. If the lesion is primarily in the insula, the standard configuration of the MCA branches will hold, and a transsylvian approach is appropriate. If the lesion is primarily of the frontal opercula and extends into the insula, the superior MCA will not likely be appreciably distorted since the superior MCA does not run in the superior insular sulcus. A combined transopercular, transsylvian approach will likely be best. If the lesion is in the dominant hemisphere, it is important to map the speech area of the operculum prior to a frontal transopercular approach.

Relationships of the Sylvian Surface of the Insula to the Operculum

The pars orbitalis overlies the accessory gyrus of the insula. Pars triangularis overlies the short insular gyrus and the insular apex. The pre- and postcentral gyrus overly the posterior superior projection of the central insular sulcus. The posterior aspect of the postcentral gyrus overlies Heschl's gyrus, and the transverse temporal gyri underlie the supramarginal gyrus.

Relationships between the sylvian surface of the insula and the internal capsule, the lenticulostriates, and the foramen of Monro Deep to the insular cortex proper lie the extreme capsule, the claustrum and the external capsule. Beneath this lie the basal ganglia, distinguished during surgery by its striate appearance. Unfortunately, this striate appearance is not much different from low-grade glioma. Medial to the basal ganglia in an obtuse angle lies the internal capsule. The genu of the internal capsule projects toward the foramen of Monro medially and is approximately 2.5 cm medial to the central insular sulcus. The anterior limb of the internal capsule projects beneath the short insular gyri, and the posterior limb of the internal capsule is only 1 cm beneath the posterior aspect of the long insular gyri.

> *Note*: It is at this level that sensorimotor deficits can inadvertently occur, either by going too deep in the resection, or more commonly, by interrupting the long perforators from the inferior branch of the MCA.

This configuration makes anterior resections less hazardous, as long as the safe mesial border, defined by the lenticulostriate arteries is not crossed. Opening the proximal sylvian fissure at the level of limen insula and looking for perforators arising from the superior aspect of M1 can identify the most lateral of the lenticulostriate arteries. If this is not possible, the lenticulostriate arteries must be carefully identified as a series of small arteries perforating the basal ganglia. Once the first of the lenticulostriate arteries is encountered, the lesional resection should stop.

A preoperative evaluation of the magnetic resonance imaging (MRI) should quickly identify the likelihood of a successful resection of the lesion. In many insular tumor cases, especially low-grade gliomas, the tumor is really just an expansion of the insular cortex, not crossing the external capsule. These cases are safe for resection. In other cases, the deeper mesial aspect of the tumor may transgress the safe borders of mesial resection: the internal capsule or the lenticulostriate arteries. In these cases, a subtotal resection of the lesion is expected. Most insular tumors are fairly well-demarcated, and restricted to safe resection zones. In some cases, the tumor may be very diffuse in nature, with ill-defined borders. These cases are most appropriate for biopsy only.

As the insula is surrounded by critical structures, the value of cortical, subcortical mapping, and awake surgery cannot be overemphasized. Once opercular mapping is done, transopercular and transsylvian resections are aided by identifying the internal capsule with subcortical mapping with a bipolar stimulator. Transsylvian resection without opercular involvement can be done with subcortical mapping alone. Furthermore, the instant feedback the surgeon has from an awake, cooperative patient can give reassurance in resections in which the lesion does not appear appreciably different from basal ganglia. It also gives the surgeon a clear stopping point if the patient develops a new mild deficit.

CHOICE OF OPERATIVE APPROACH

As mentioned, operative approaches to the insula include the transsylvian fissure and transcortical approaches. The choice of approach depends on a number of preoperative and intraoperative factors.

On preoperative evaluation, the MRI and a thorough understanding of the anatomical relationship of the tumor to the surrounding anatomy and vasculature is the key. Lesions that are small, confined to the insula with clear borders may be resected through the transsylvian approach regardless of location within the insula due to the need for a small operative approach. However, larger lesions especially when involving the posterosuperior insula may require a combined approach due to a large amount of retraction on the frontal and temporal opercula if a pure transsylvian approach is chosen. This can lead to direct injuries from retraction or compression of the sylvian vein.

In cases where the lesion has encompassed part of the frontal or parietal opercula, a transcortical approach can be straight forward. Previously eloquent language, motor, or sensory area may have been replaced by pathology and no longer deemed eloquent. The commitment to a transcortical approach is often made intraoperatively after mapping is done. Constant communication with an awake patient is useful in ensuring neurological function is preserved.

Anteriorly in the frontal operculum on the dominant side, the motor speech "Broca's" areas, classically known as Brodmann's areas 44 and 45 are seen in the posterior half of pars opercularis and pars triangularis. Therefore, with careful mapping, the pars orbitalis and the anterior pars opercularis may be resected to provide an enhanced operative window to the anterior insula. The next opercular structure on superiorly is the precentral gyrus, specifically the motor face region. Resection of this area does lead to immediate postoperative contralateral facial paresis, but if the resection only involves the face motor region, recovery is usually excellent with return of function seen around 6 weeks to 3 months after surgery. Resection of the opercular postcentral gyrus leads to contralateral somatosensory loss of the face region. Resection posterior to the postcentral gyrus is not needed in approaches to the posterior insula. On the temporal opercular side, mapping of the superior temporal gyrus is the key to identifying positive language areas that may limit cortical resection. Heschl's gyrus receives bilateral inputs from the inferior colliculi and medical geniculate bodies. Therefore, unilateral resection of Heschl's gyrus does not cause perceptible loss of auditory function. Cortical resection posterior to Heschl's gyrus or angular gyrus should not be performed due to risk of language deficit. Lastly, if a transcortical approach involving the Heschl's gyrus is chosen, extensive subcortical mapping is critical on the dominant side. Fibers of arcuate and middle longitudinal fasciculi run medial to this area and can be distorted by the lesion.

CASE 1: LEFT ANTEROSUPERIOR INSULAR LOW-GRADE GLIOMA

History

A 31-year-old right-handed female with focal right hand seizure and identified nonenhancing lesion involving the left anterior superior insula encroaching upon the claustrum and external capsule.

Magnetic resonance imaging (MRI) (Figs. 5.1A and B) of the brain revealed a nonenhancing lesion involving the left anterior insula extending superiorly to the centrum semiovale and

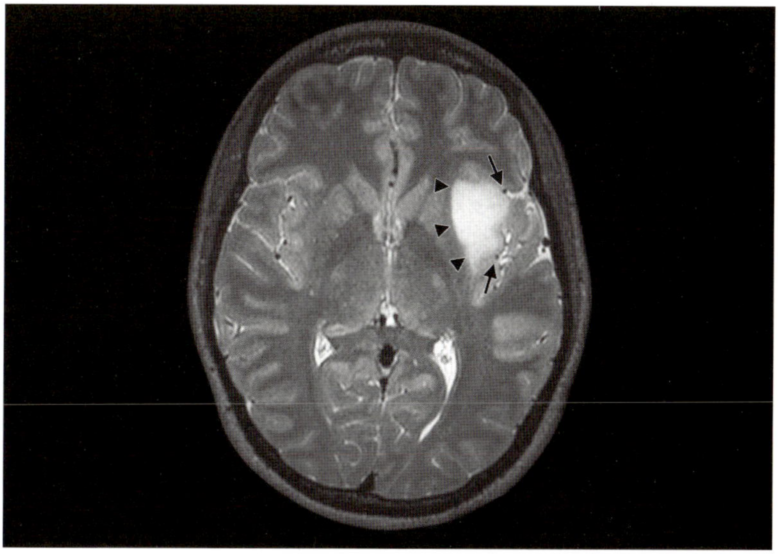

Fig. 5.1A: Preoperative MRI of brain. T2-weighted (T2W) axial image with the left insular hyperintense lesion seen. The M2 branches bordering the lesion are visible (arrows). The medial border of the tumor (arrowheads) approaches and causes mass effect upon the putamen.

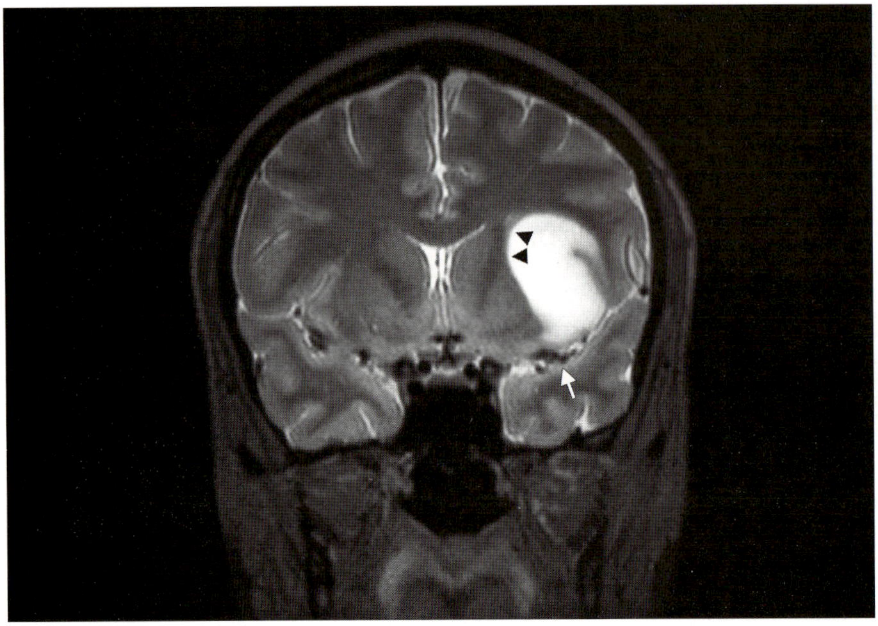

Fig. 5.1B: T2W coronal image of the same lesion demonstrating the superior extension of the tumor. Note the extremely close relationship between the superior-medial border of the tumor and internal capsule (arrowheads). The candelabra of early M2 branches (arrow) are seen inferior to the bulk of tumor.

medially to the external capsule. There was no enhancement suggesting a likely low-grade nature.

Given the dominant side and anterior superior location of the lesion, an awake craniotomy with cortical and subcortical mapping via a transsylvian approach was planned.

Surgery (Fig. 5.2)

After dural opening, the sylvian fissure was dissected anteriorly down to the carotid artery and posteriorly to the precentral gyrus. The M1 and lenticulostriates were interior to the lesion as expected. Middle cerebral artery (MCA) bifurcation was noted and both M2 branches were followed and carefully dissected.

The corticotomy plane was chosen between the two M2 branches and upon entering the insula tumor-like tissue was encountered. Early biopsy was sent confirming low-grade glioma as the diagnosis. The tumor was debulked to allow for relaxation and inferior migration of superior components in order to reduce the need for retraction of the frontal operculum.

Using continuous motor examinations and subcortical mapping, resection continued superiorly and medially until no further abnormal tissue was seen under the microscope (Figs. 5.3A and B).

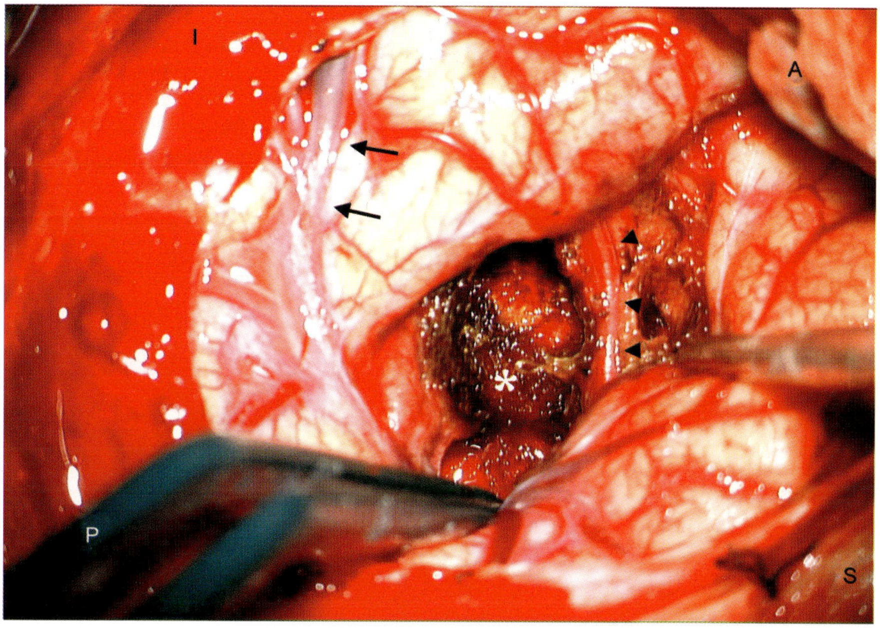

Fig. 5.2: Intraoperative photograph demonstrating the resection cavity. The sylvian fissure has been divided and the frontal operculum retracted. The resection cavity within the insula can be readily seen (star). The superior branch of M2 is visible (arrowheads). The vein of Labbé is shown by arrows.

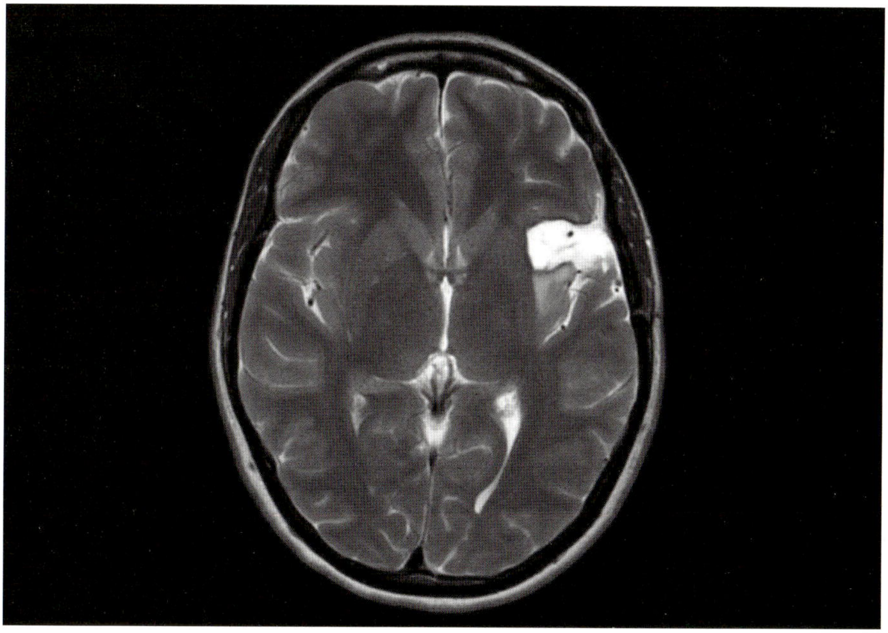

Fig. 5.3A: Postoperative MRI of brain obtained 6 months after resection. Axial T2-weighted (T2W).

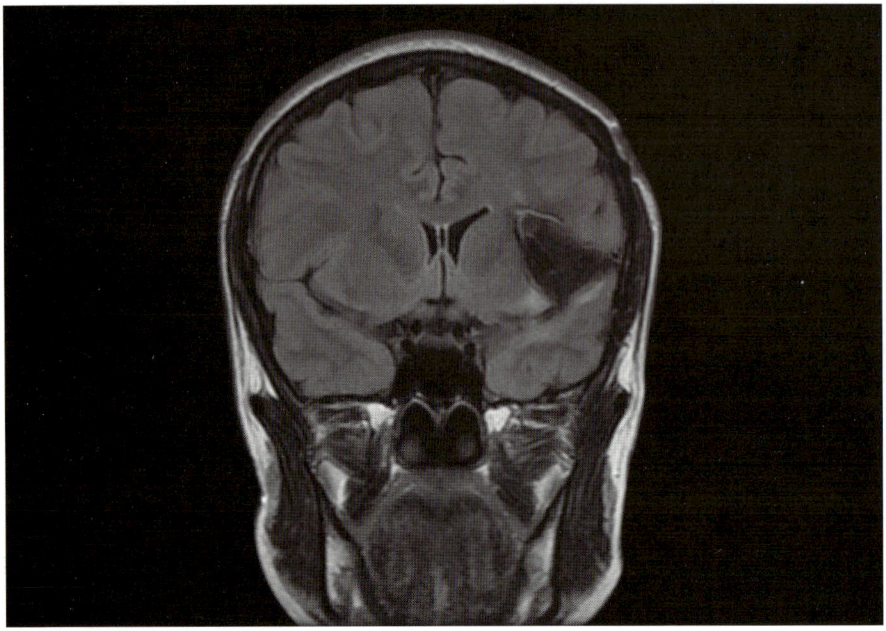

Fig. 5.3B: Coronal fast fluid-attenuated inversion recovery (FLAIR) images demonstrating the resection cavity.

CASE 2: LEFT INSULAR-SUBFRONTAL LOW-GRADE GLIOMA; COMBINED TRANSSYLVIAN/SUBFRONTAL-TRANSCORTICAL APPROACH

History

A 28-year-old right-handed male with history of refractory seizures who was found to have a large left sided lesion involving the frontal and temporal lobe as well as the insula.

Magnetic resonance imaging was revealing of a large nonenhancing mass encompassing the subfrontal area extending anteromedially to the interhemispheric fissure. The mid-portion of the mass engulfed the insula and temporal stem, abutting the amygdala. The interior border of the lesion was marked by the lenticulostriate arteries arising from the M1 (Figs. 5.4A to C).

Given the dominant side and the multilobar configuration, an awake craniotomy using a combined subfrontal, transcortical and a transsylvian insular approach was planned.

Surgery (Figs. 5.5 and 5.6)

After dural opening, mapping ensued revealing positive language arrest upon stimulation of the pars opercularis. Mapping was negative in the pars triangularis area and the superior temporal gyrus. As such the frontal lobe was entered through a subfrontal, trans-pars orbitalis approach and tumor was readily seen. Debulking was performed, leading to brain relaxation. Resection was carried medially until the interhemispheric fissure.

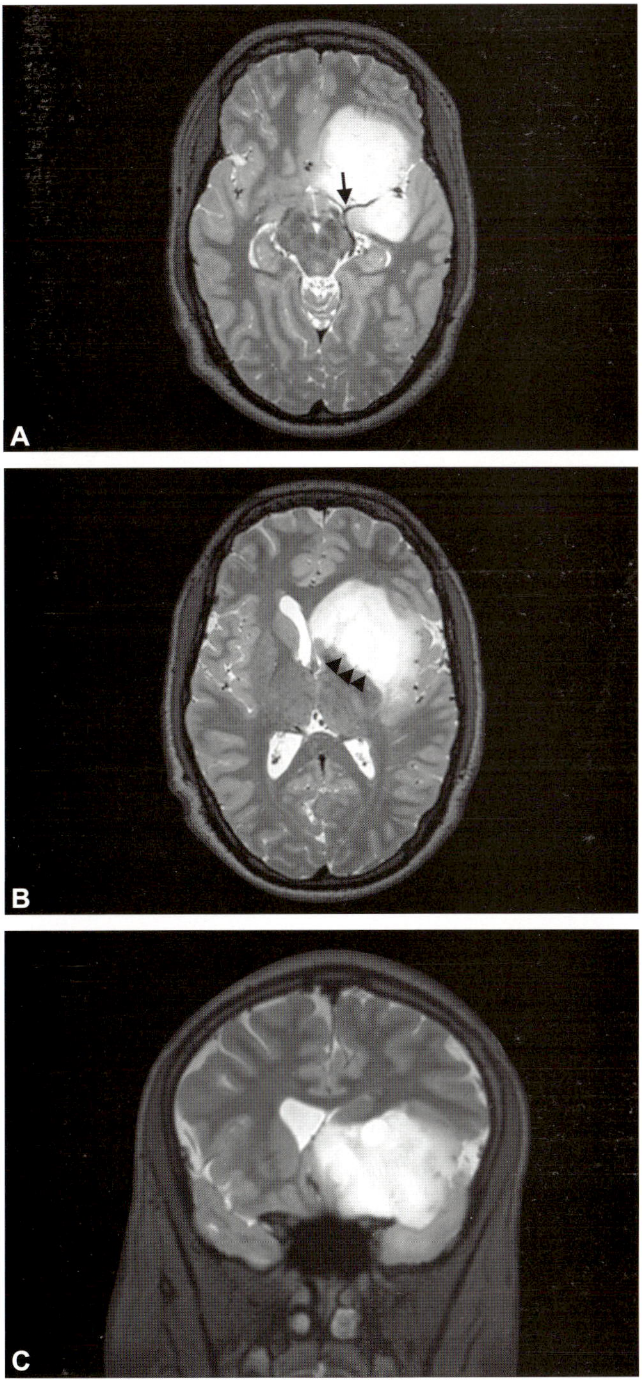

Figs. 5.4A to C: Preoperative MRI of brain. (A and B) Axial T2-weighted (T2W)) images at the level of the carotid bifurcation (A) (arrow) and foramen of Monro (B) demonstrating the extent of tumor borders. Note the draping of lenticulostriate arteries medially (arrowheads). (C) Coronal T2W image showing the medial extension involving the frontal horn and interhemispheric fissure.

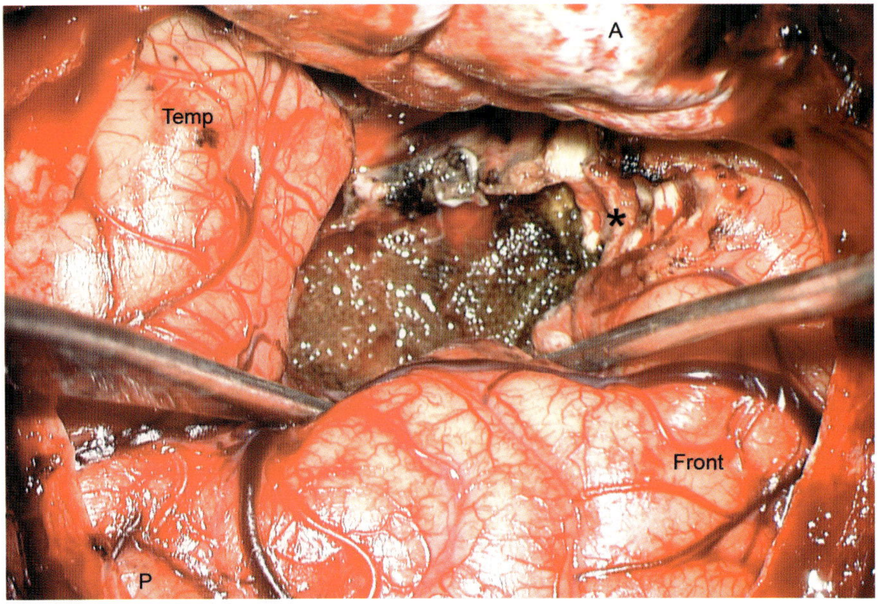

Fig. 5.5: Intraoperative photograph demonstrating the resection cavity. The sylvian fissure has been divided and retracted. The subfrontal, trans-pars orbitalis approach (star) is visible.
(A: Anterior; P: Posterior).

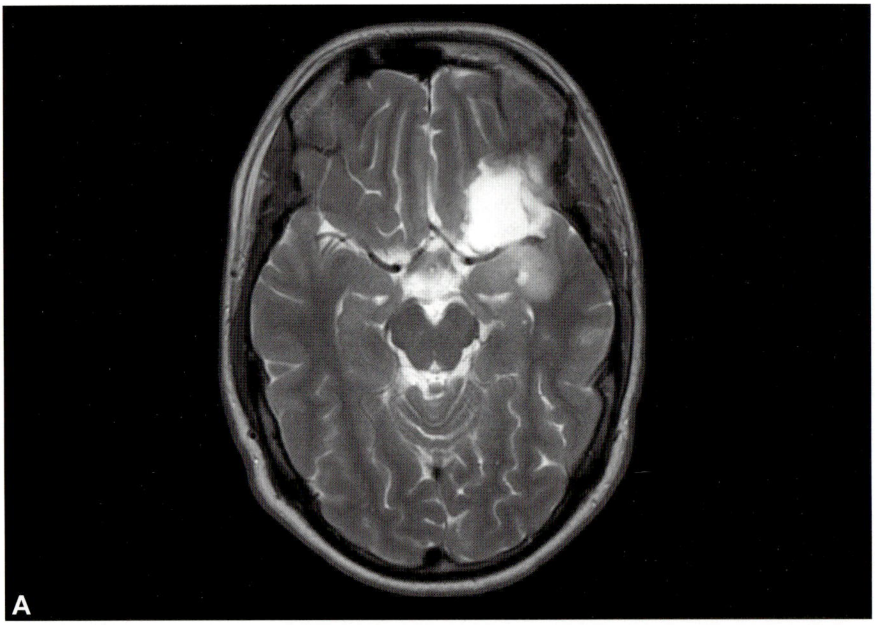

Fig. 5.6A: Postoperative MRI of brain obtained 6 months after resection.

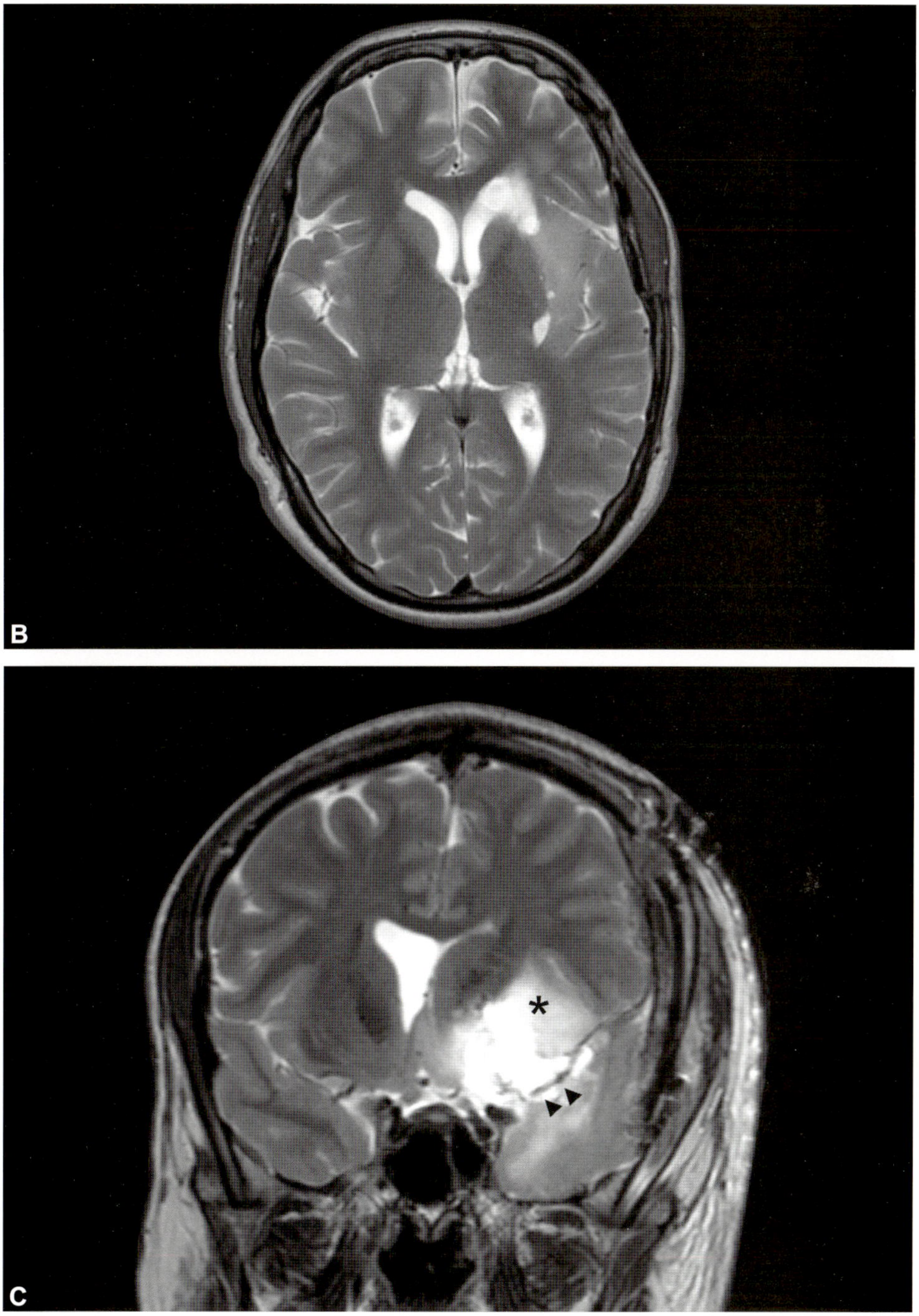

Figs. 5.6B and C: (B) Corresponding axial images demonstrating large partial resection. (C) Coronal corresponding image shows the reanimation of basal ganglia. Note the skeletonized M1 (arrowheads) and the signal abnormality in the area shown (star) where resection stopped due to speech dysarthria.

Next, the sylvian fissure was dissected to expose the anterior insula and temporal stem. Further debulking of tumor was performed with continuous contralateral motor and speech examinations. As resection approached the insula and medial structures, subcortical mapping was done repeatedly, until normal looking tissue was encountered. During dissection of the posteromedial elements of tumor, patient began to exhibit dysarthria and word finding difficulties and as such resection stopped.

Postoperatively, the patient recovered normal speech and had no other neurologic deficits.

CASE 3: LEFT POSTERIOR INSULA CAVERNOMA (TRANSSYLVIAN APPROACH)

History

A 23-year-old right-handed male with history of focal sensory seizures involving the right face, arm and leg. CT found a left insular mass with recent hemorrhage.

Magnetic resonance imaging revealed a "popcorn" lesion involving the posterior long gyrus of the insula with hemosiderin signal and surrounding signal change involving the opercular segment of the postcentral gyrus (Figs. 5.7A to C). Angiogram was negative for an occult vascular malformation.

After review of the images, in light of the smaller size of the lesion, a transsylvian approach to the insula was chosen as the corridor with an awake craniotomy.

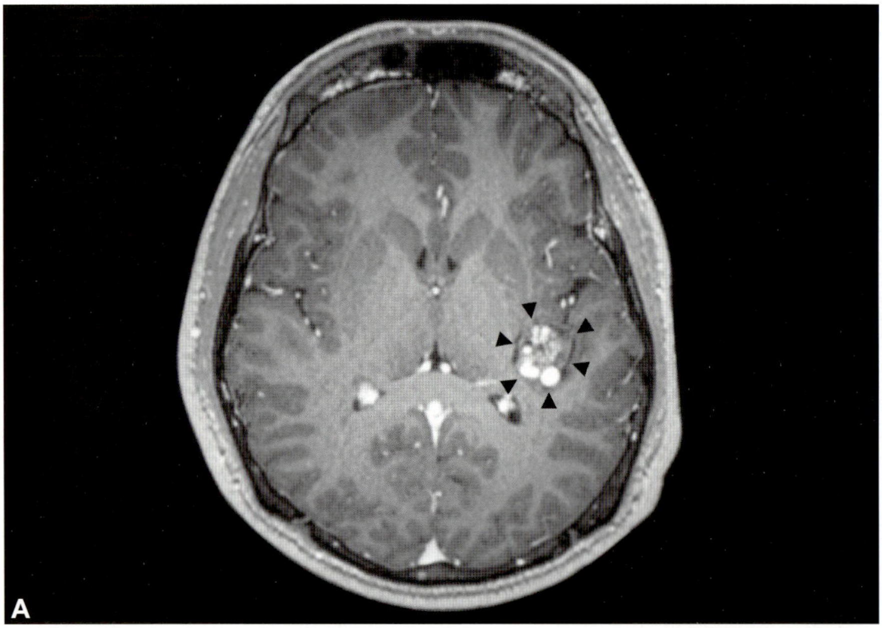

Fig. 5.7A: Preoperative MRI of brain. Axial T1-weighted (T1W) postcontrast image demonstrating the enhancing lesion along the posterior insula (arrowheads).

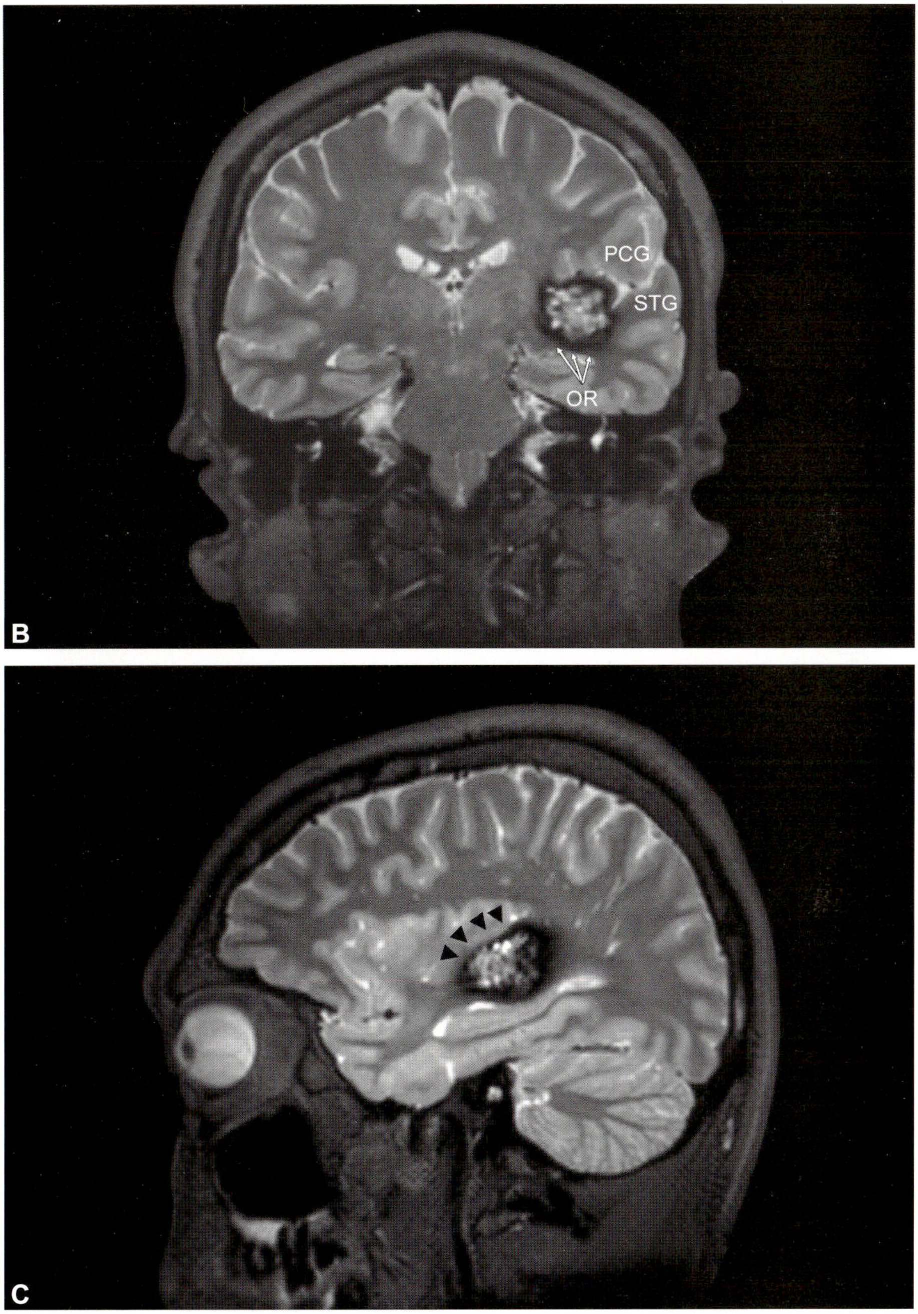

Figs. 5.7B and C: (B) Coronal T2W image reveals the surrounding anatomy. The sylvian fissure corridor is abutted by the postcentral gyrus (PCG) and the superior temporal gyrus (STG). Note the intimate inferior association of the lesion with the optic radiation fibers (arrows, OR) running on the roof of temporal horn. (C) Sagittal T2W image demonstrates the location of the lesion along the posterior long gyrus of the insula (arrowheads).

Surgery (Figs. 5.8 A to D)

After dural opening, mapping localized the pre- and postcentral gyri. Superior temporal gyrus mapping did not reveal any positive language findings. Angular gyrus was mapped with language slowing.

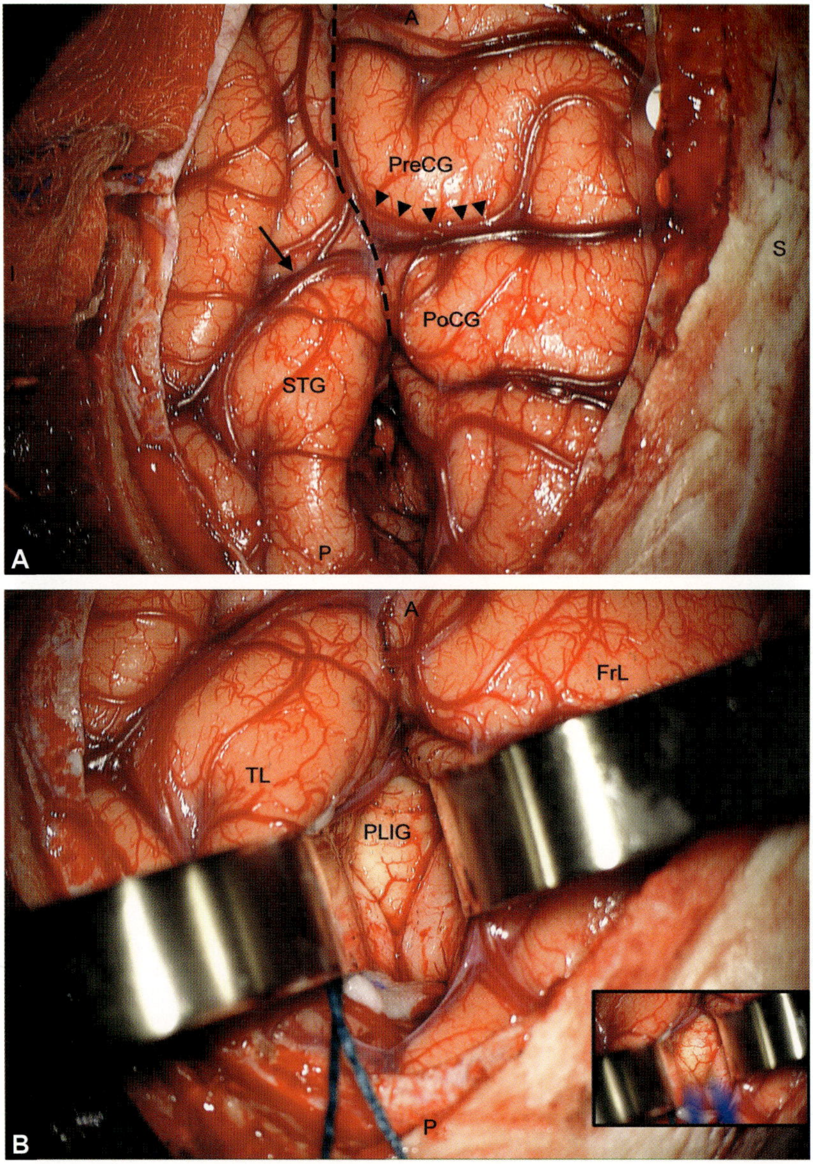

Figs. 5.8A and B: Intraoperative photographs demonstrating the relevant anatomy. (A) The sylvian fissure (dotted line) has been opened to expose the long insular gyri. (B) The frontal (FrL) and temporal (TL) lobes have been retracted to reveal the posterior long insular gyrus (PLIG) (PreCG: Precentral gyrus; PoCG: Postcentral gyrus; STG: Superior temporal gyrus; A: Anterior; S: Superior; I: Inferior; P: Posterior: Arrowheads: Central artery; arrow: Heschl's gyrus).

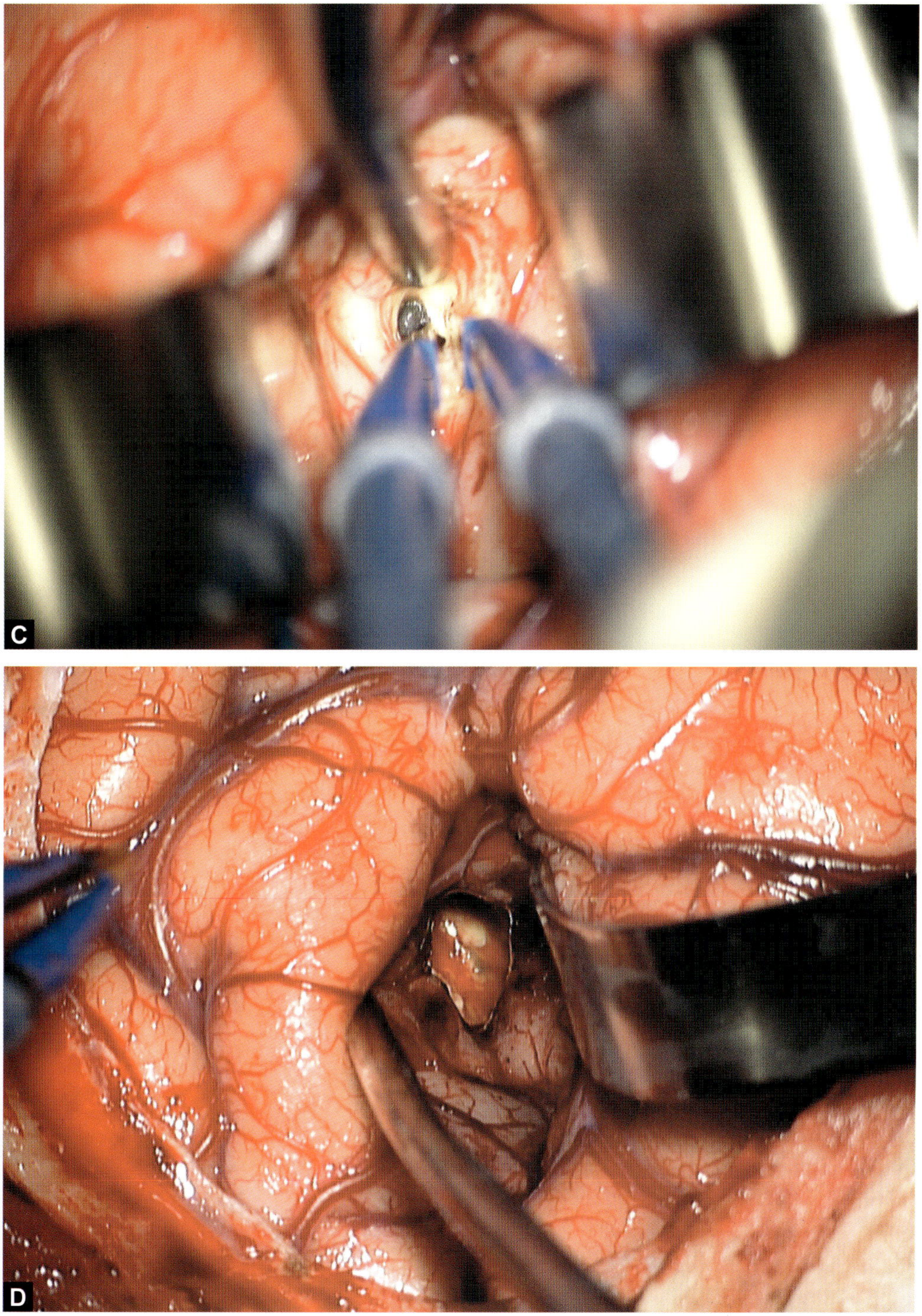

Figs. 5.8C and D: (C) The posterior long insular gyrus has been opened revealing the cavernous malformation. (D) Resection cavity after complete removal of the cavernous malformation.

The sylvian fissure was subsequently opened with meticulous care taken to preserve the sylvian vein. Distal M2 and M3 branches were gently retracted and the posterior long gyrus of the insula was exposed. After retraction of the frontal and temporal opercula, the insular gyrus was mapped by stimulation without any positive findings. As such, it was entered via a corticotomy and the cavernous malformation was resected en-bloc with continuous communication with the patient. Care was taken during medial resection as to not injure the traversing arcuate and middle longitudinal fasciculi.

The patient had no postoperative difficulties and was discharged home on day 2 (Figs. 5.9A and B).

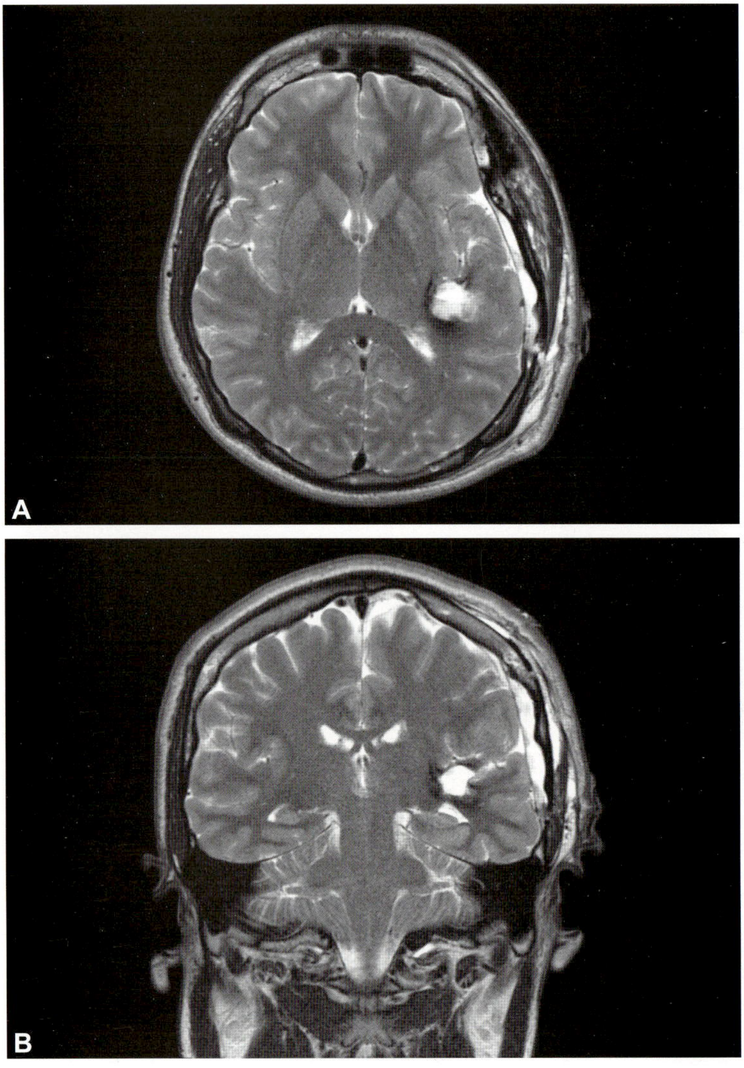

Figs. 5.9A and B: Postoperative MRI of brain. (A) Axial T2-weighted (T2W) image and (B) Coronal T2W images demonstrate the resection cavity.

CHAPTER

6

Occipital Interhemispheric Approach to Limbic Tumors

Vikas K Parmar, Ilhan Aydin, Emel Avci, Mustafa K Baskaya

INTRODUCTION

"Occipital" derives from Latin *occiput*, a combination of *ob* meaning "against, behind", and *caput* meaning "head". The occipital lobe carries the primary and secondary visual cortex, Brodmann areas 17 and 18, 19, respectively. The interhemispheric fissure between the right and the left occipital poles can provide a corridor favorable for specific tumors and vascular malformations. In this chapter we will discuss the basic and surgical anatomy, the relative indications, details of the surgical approach, risks and pitfalls, and a few case illustrations of the posterior interhemispheric or occipital interhemispheric approach to limbic tumor pathology.

HISTORY

Georges Guillain, a famous French neurologist, first described of a 52-year-old male who complained of headache and demonstrated marked memory disturbances. *The first symptoms had shown themselves in February, 1920. The patient died in October 1920, and evolution relatively rapid for cerebral tumors. Necropsy examination confirmed the diagnosis of tumor of the splenium.*[1]

Such pathology is now best treated surgically with the occipital interhemispheric approach with or without a transtentorial component. This was first described by Horrax in 1937 and had since been modified by Poppen and by Jamieson in 1960s and 1970s, respectively.[2-5] Now, the occipital interhemispheric approach has become the workhorse for various posterior limbic pathologies.

ANATOMY

The occipital lobe carries the primary and the secondary visual cortex. The primary visual cortex, V1 or Brodmann area 17, is located on the walls and the floors of the calcarine sulcus; the macula is represented by the posterior third of the calcarine cortex.

The surface anatomy of the occipital lobe is often overlooked. The limits of the occipital lobe can be demarcated medially with the parietal-occipital sulcus; laterally, by an imaginary line of which the parietal-occipital sulcus meets the preoccipital notch. The calcarine sulcus is another major sulcus in the occipital lobe that separates the cuneus from the lingual gyrus. The cuneus gyrus is located along the medial surface, between the parietal-occipital sulcus and the calcarine sulcus. The lingual gyrus lies along the tentorial surface of the occipital lobe and is inferior to the calcarine sulcus. The fusiform gyrus is just inferior and medial to the lingual gyrus and is separated from the lingual gyrus by the collateral sulcus.[6]

There are various white matter fiber tracts going to the occipital lobe that neurosurgeons should be aware of. The lateral geniculate body itself gives off geniculocalcarine fibers, also known as the optic radiation. The temporal loop or Meyer's loop follows the inferior longitudinal fasciculus to the occipital pole. The inferior longitudinal fasciculus runs along the U fibers of the cortical occipital lobe. The lateral geniculate body also gives off parietal geniculocalcarine fibers that pass close to the outer wall of the lateral ventricles to the calcarine sulcus. It does also have output pathway called the corticofugal fibers back to the superior colliculus and lateral geniculate body. Other fiber tracts to be wary of include those that pass through the splenium of the corpus callosum, also known as the forceps major, which delineated along the medial aspect of the posterior wall of the lateral ventricle. The forceps major allows communication between the right and left occipital lobes.

Knowledge of the ventricular anatomy around the occipital lobe is imperative, especially in cases where extra brain relaxation is needed and there is a potential need for a parietal occipital external ventricular drain placement. In the depths of the occipital lobe the occipital horns of the lateral ventricles can be found. The walls of the occipital horn can be defined by the tapetum, fibers that form the splenium of the corpus callosum forming the roof and lateral wall. The collateral eminence, or the indentation of the collateral sulcus on the lateral ventricle, defines the floor. The calcar avis, or the deepest aspect of the calcarine sulcus, defines the medial wall. The occipital horn ends anteriorly as the parieto-occipital sulcus emerges. This anatomy is crucial in the posterior interhemispheric fissure; if the surgeon were to penetrate the ventricle through this approach, he or she should be considered at the level of the precuneus.[7]

One must have a very firm grasp of the vascular anatomy in this region to be successful with the posterior occipital interhemispheric approach. The major and obvious consideration is that of opening over the torcula, the inferior portion of the superior sagittal sinus, the occipital sinus and both transverse sinuses. Unlike the parietal-occipital interhemispheric approach, the occipital interhemispheric approach has no bridging draining veins into the sagittal sinus. As one proceeds down the falx-occipital fissure, the internal occipital veins, which drain into the vein of Galen, can be found. Even deeper lies the arachnoid of the quadrigeminal cistern and its vascular contents: ipsilateral basal vein of Rosenthal, posterior medial choroidal artery, and the posterior cerebral artery (PCA) P3 and P4 segment. The P3 segment of posterior cerebral artery travels posteriorly from the ambient cistern into the quadrigeminal cistern. The medial posterior choroidal artery typically begins from the P1 or P2 segment through the ambient cistern, continues inferior and medial to the PCA into the quadrigeminal cistern. The lateral posterior choroidal arteries arise typically from the second segment of the PCA at the posterior portion edge of the ambient cistern and courses laterally along the parahippocampal gyrus, pierces through the choroidal fissure into the temporal horn of the ventricle. The anterior choroidal artery also courses laterally and enters the ventricle at the inferior choroidal point.

Table 6.1: Relative indications and contraindications.

Relative indications	*Relative contraindications*
Splenium tumors	Right hemianopsia
Occipital lobe tumors	Tumors primarily infratentorial
Posterior falcine tumors	Tumors primarily parietal
Pineal region tumors	
Posterior incisor tumors	
Posterior mesial temporal tumors	
Intraventricular trigone tumors	

Of note, in the occipital interhemispheric approach, typically the anterior choroidal artery (AChA) and the lateral posterior choroidal artery (PChA) are inaccessible; whereas, the distal medial PChA could be accessed. The localization of nearby anatomy regardless is important.[8]

INDICATIONS/CONTRAINDICATIONS FOR APPROACH

In 1920, Georges Guillain described the symptomatology of splenial tumors.

1. *Signs of intracranial hypertension, with vomiting, headache, and sometimes pupillary stasis.*
2. *Mental symptoms characterized by amnesia, bizarre acts and attitudes, emotional indiffe-rence, disorientation, and sometimes by mental confusion.*
3. *Frequent presence of paralyses, contractures, and bilateral hypertonias.*[1]

Even today, patients who present with pathology of the posterior limbic system (splenium, posterior cingulate gyrus) often present with very similar symptoms as described in 1920. Patients with occipital lobe tumors often present with visual auras or hallucinations, headaches, general mental impairment, or transient/progressive changes in vision.[9] Pineal region tumors can present with endocrine abnormalities, Parinaud's syndrome, or obstructive hydrocephalus. Regardless of the location of the mass, symptomatic lesions in or near the posterior limbic system are indications for an occipital interhemispheric approach. These relative indications are summarized in Table 6.1. The pathologies as determined by magnetic resonance imaging (MRI) particularly amendable for resection via an occipital interhemispheric approach include lesions of the posterior cingulate gyrus, posterior portion of the parahippocampal gyrus and lingual gyrus, tumors of the splenium of the corpus callosum, tumors directly in the occipital lobe along the falx, lesions originating from the posterior falx or posterior incisor, posterior mesial temporal lobe, intraventricular tumors of the trigone or posterior horns, and midline tumors of the pineal region.[10-15]

Relative contraindications for pursing the posterior occipital interhemispheric approach are also summarized in Table 6.1. Sectioning the splenium can interrupt the transfer of visual information from nondominant hemispheres to the dominant hemisphere. A relative contraindication would be preoperative right hemianopsia as the patient would only have left visual fields and right occipital lobe intact. As such separating the splenium would cause disconnection between the two. Tumors that are primarily infratentorial may be better candidates for the supracerebellar infratentorial approach. However, Figueiredo et al. does describe in an anatomical study that the anatomy visualized is similar for the occipital interhemispheric and the infratentorial supracerebellar approach.[8] Also, deep parietal tumors of which the shortest distance from cortex to tumor is more favorable for a posterior parietal interhemispheric approach should typically not be attempted with an occipital interhemispheric approach.

Main limitation of this approach is the need for retraction of the medial, interhemispheric surface of the occipital lobe, which puts pressure on the calcarine visual cortex. Pathology that is more parietal and more along the posterior cingulate gyrus rather than splenium are apt for a posterior parietal interhemispheric approach. This approach does often have bridging veins that can bleed if one is not careful in dural opening. Also, brain relaxation via releasing cerebrospinal fluid in nearby cisterns is often not possible with the posterior parietal interhemispheric approach.

In contrast, the posterior occipital interhemispheric approach has few to no bridging veins in reference to the sagittal sinus. However, special attention should be taken regarding the bridging veins around the vein of Galen. Main advantage of the occipital interhemispheric approach is that it allows wide exposure of lesions that extend bilaterally or from the posterior parahippocampal gyrus extending to the cingulate gyrus via isthmus as demonstrated in Figures 6.1A to F and 6.2A to D. There is also easy access to blood supply particularly to the medial posterior choroidal arteries, the posterior pericallosal arteries, and the distal posterior cerebral arteries (parieto-occipital branches).

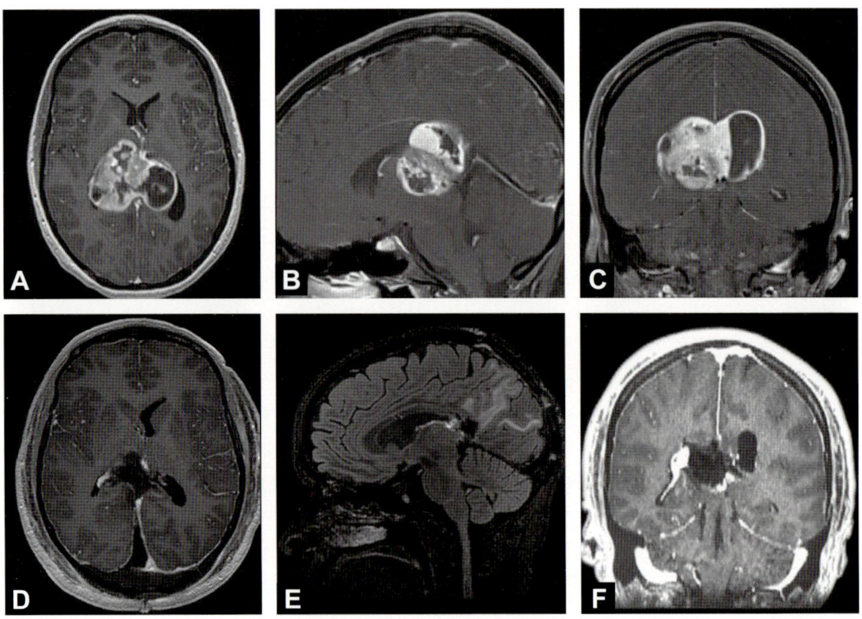

Figs. 6.1A to F: Magnetic resonance imaging (MRI) of a 26-year-old female who presented with memory problems and personality changes. Preoperative (A) axial T1, (B) sagittal T1, (C) coronal T1 postcontrast, MRIs show very large heterogeneously enhancing mass lesion extending from the right thalamus to the posterior cingulate gyrus. Postoperative (D) axial T1, (E) coronal T1 postcontrast and (F) T2 flair-cube postcontrast MRI, show gross total resection after occipital interhemispheric approach has been utilized.

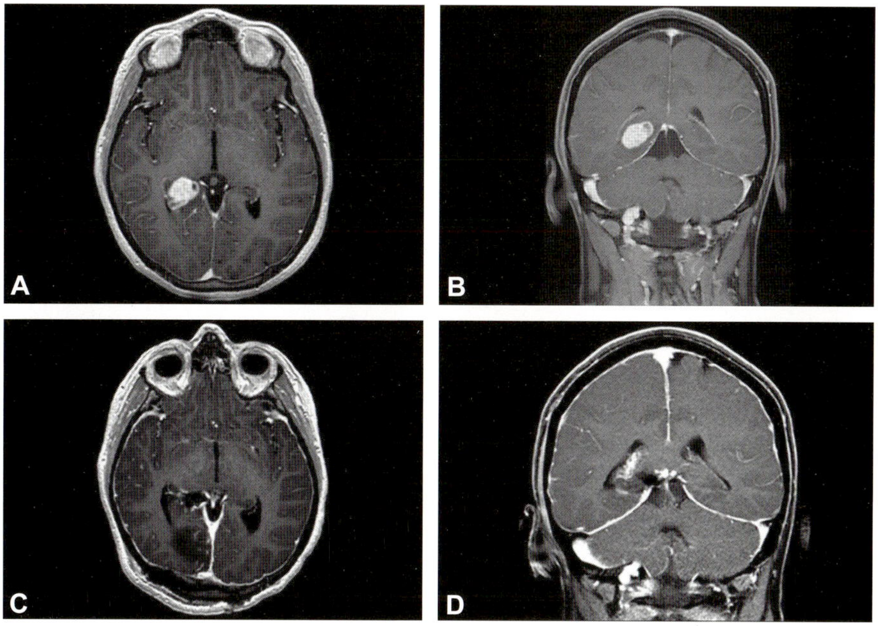

Figs. 6.2A to D: Magnetic resonance imaging (MRI) of a 40-year-old female with generalized seizures. Preoperative (A) axial T1 and (B) coronal T1 postcontrast MRIs show contrast enhancing mass lesion in the posterior parahippocampus and arachnoid cyst in the quadrigeminal cistern. Postoperative (C) axial T1 and (D) coronal T1 postcontrast MRIs show gross total resection after occipital interhemispheric approach has been utilized.

Details of Surgical Approach

For our occipital interhemispheric approach, brain relaxation is of the utmost importance as the occipital lobe tends not to be forgiving in regards to retraction.[16] As such, the surgery begins with a lumbar drain placement at the beginning of the case. After lumbar drain placement, that patient is carefully placed in the Mayfield pin head holder and then turned prone onto the operative table with Bardeen chest and hip rolls.

Another variation in position is the three-fourths prone position. The legs are flexed with a pillow between them and elevated to facilitate venous return, and the patient is strapped down so that the table can be rotated during the procedure to improve exposure when appropriate. The three-fourths prone position is essentially an extension of the lateral position, except that the head is at an oblique 45° angle. Unlike the prone position, the nondominant hemisphere in the three-fourths prone is easily retracted with the help of gravity. Surgeon fatigue is reduced. Axillary roll often is not even needed under the patient's right axilla with the right arm supported with an arm board.[17]

Neuronavigation is then registered to plan out the midline incision as well as site for a ventriculostomy if needed during the case. Three incisions can be utilized for this approach: midline, straight vertical incision, U-shaped incision, or curvilinear, hockey-stick incision (Figs. 6.3A and B). Frequently a U-shaped incision is used to reflect a myocutaneous flap

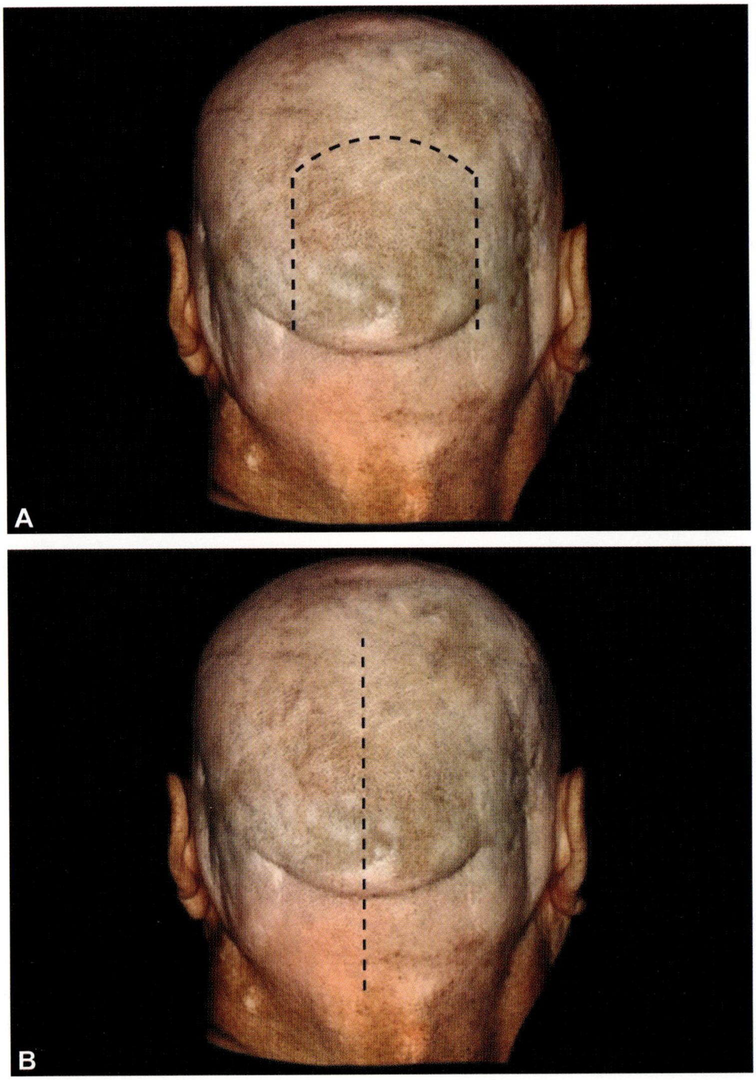

Figs. 6.3A and B: Commonly used skin incisions are demonstrated in cadaveric dissections. (A) Reverse U-shaped incision crossing the midline. (B) Long vertical straight incision is used to cross midline sagittal sinus.

inferiorly as shown in Figure 6.4. The periosteal layer is also elevated and the craniotomy should be carefully planned with neuronavigation. The sagittal sinus, the torcula, tentorium/transverse sinuses, and bridging veins should all be marked. The medial, lateral, superior, and inferior edges of the tumor should also be considered to guarantee an adequate operative corridor. Burr holes are then placed strategically. We typically opt to place six burr holes: two burr holes superior and lateral off the sagittal sinus, two burr holes inferior (just above the level of the transverse sinus) and lateral off the sagittal sinus, and two burr holes laterally on each side to expand the craniotomy

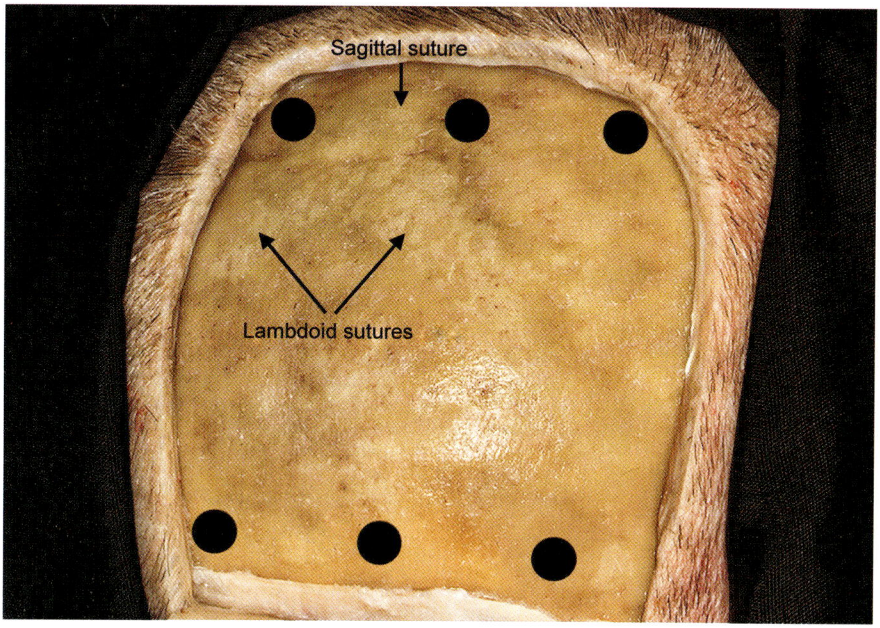

Fig. 6.4: Placement of burr holes for occipital interhemispheric approach in cadaveric dissection. Burr holes are placed either side of the sagittal sinus superiorly and inferiorly to safety elevate the dura off the sinus. Burr holes just above the level of the transverse sinus, and burr holes laterally on each side to expand the craniotomy. Additional burr holes are placed just above the transverse sinus to accomplish lowest exposure possible towards the tentorium.

(Fig. 6.4). Figure 6.5A depicts the operative field after craniotomy. Prior to dural opening, mannitol can be useful for relaxing the brain and minimizing the risk for hemianopia from excessive occipital lobe retraction. We then use a scalpel to incise the dura on the left side out laterally and approximately 2 cm off midline and then use Metzenbaum scissors to further extend the dural opening paralleling the sagittal sinus as shown in Figure 6.5B and at the very ends of the craniotomy turning until it comes just to the sagittal sinus both anteriorly and posteriorly. One should be wary of draining veins at this point as Neurolon sutures are used to retract the dura medially.

At this point, careful dissection along the falx and along the occipital and parietal lobes is performed as demonstrated in Figure 6.6. The straight sinus and the superior sagittal sinus should be well appreciated. The dissection is carried deeper until the splenium and the regional anatomy is encountered (Figs. 6.7A and B). Again, to reiterate, it is key to avoid retraction on the occipital lobe. Medial occipital lobe can be protected with paddies and a retractor can be placed over the falx for exposure. The inferior sagittal sinus and falx can be divided to facilitate further falcine retraction. Often there is bleeding seen on the inferior edge of the falx, and this can be controlled with a combination of bipolar coagulation and Gelfoam. At all times, the location of the straight sinus should be identified at the falcotentorial junction and can be done so by intraoperative Doppler. The tumor is then visualized often at this point and as such dissection in all directions around the tumor is done until relatively normal-appearing

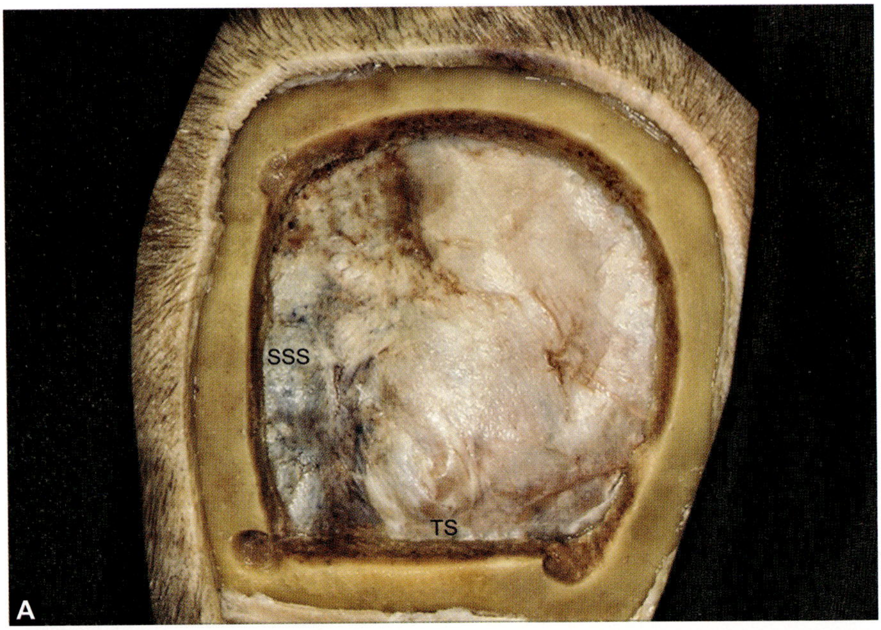

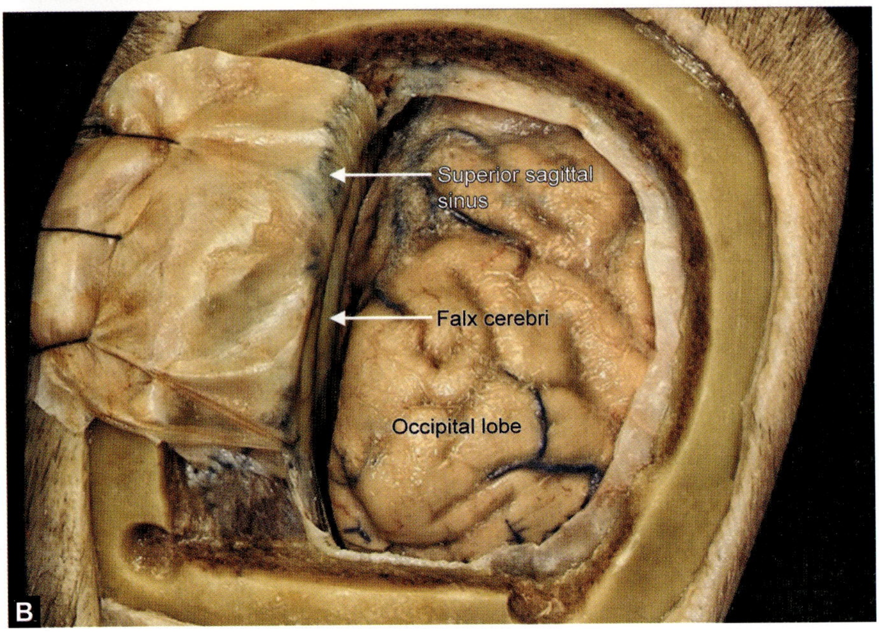

Figs. 6.5A and B: (A) Occipital craniotomy crossing the superior sagittal sinus (SSS) above the transverse sinus (TS). (B) The dural opening should parallel the sagittal sinus and should turn at the very ends of the craniotomy until it comes just to the sagittal sinus both anteriorly and posteriorly. One should be aware of draining veins as the dura is retracted medially.

tissue is reached. The contents of the quadrigeminal cistern must be visualized and the deep venous anatomy must always be appreciated when proceeding with tumor resection.

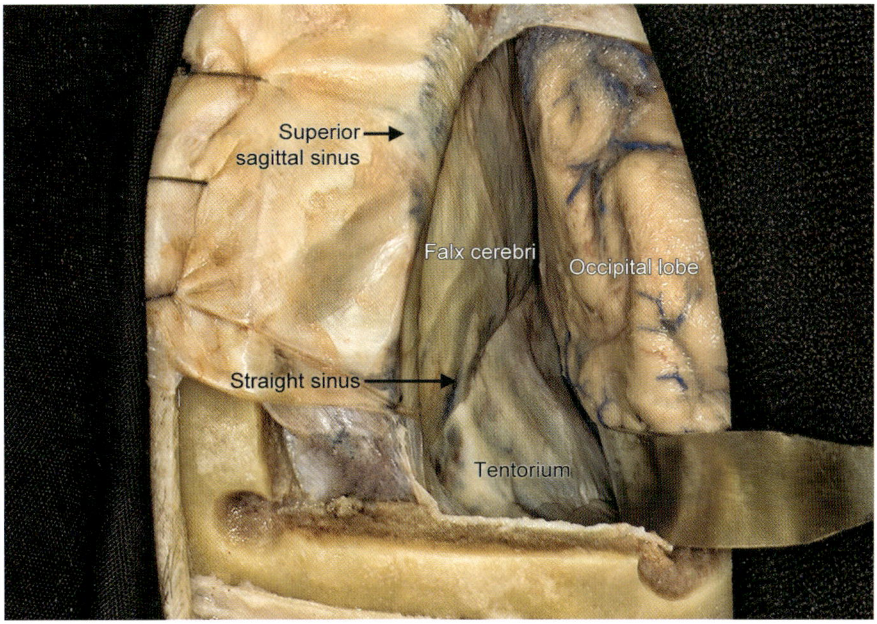

Fig. 6.6: Interhemispheric dissection: Dissection along the falx and the occipital lobe should reveal the straight sinus and the tentorium.

The pineal gland is just inferior to the venous complex of the quadrigeminal cistern; the pulvinar region of the thalamus is just deep and lateral to the splenium (Fig. 6.8). Care must be taken in regards to the branches of the PCA arising from the quadrigeminal cistern as depicted in Figure 6.8. If the ventricle is penetrated we opt to use Gelfoam to keep blood from getting into the ventricle. In the meantime during tumor resection, stealth neuronavigation is used repeatedly to identify the limits of the resection. If needed, the tentorium can be incised and reflected laterally for a wider operative corridor to a specific pathology. If doing so, the location of the straight sinus must be redemonstrated. Also, one must be wary of the trochlear nerve, which runs along the posterior incisor. Of note, Yasargil describes that to access intraventricular pathology through this approach an incision in the precuneus gyrus can be performed; this preserves the integrity of the optic radiations.[18] After gross total resection we turn our attention to closure and meticulous hemostasis. We line the resection bed with surgicel and copiously irrigate the resection bed until the saline is clear. The dura is closed with interrupted Neurolon sutures. We cover the dura with surgicel and then plate the bone back into position.

RISKS AND PITFALLS

As with every surgical approach, the occipital interhemispheric approach has its own specific risks. First, over retraction of the occipital lobe can precipitate homonymous hemianopsia. This can be avoided by using adequate brain relaxation techniques, retractors on the falx, and avoidance of retractors on medial occipital lobe.

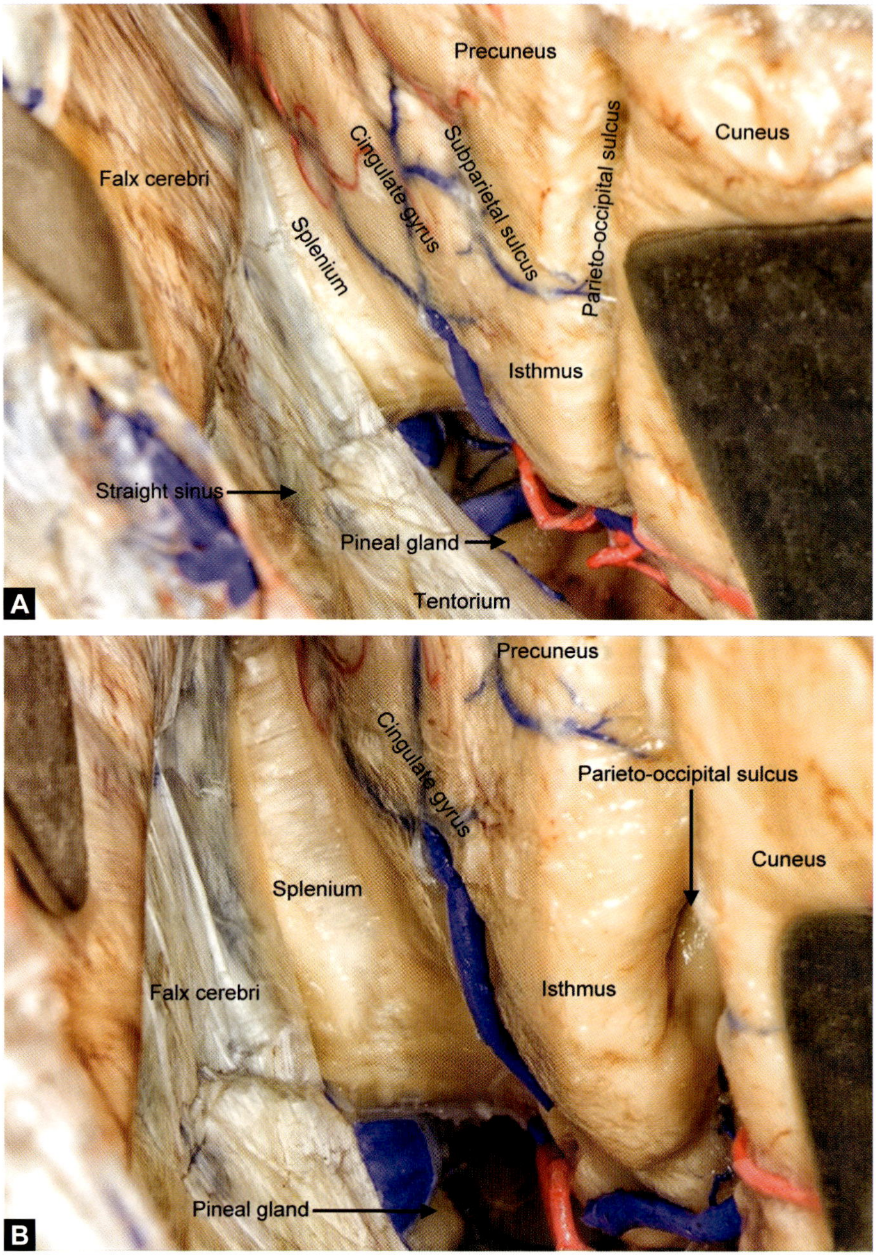

Figs. 6.7A and B: (A) At the depths of the dissection, the splenium is encountered. Above this is the cingulate gyrus. Even more superficial is the precuneus and cuneus, separated by the parieto-occipital sulcus. The pineal gland can also be visualized as one approaches the quadrigeminal cistern. (B) In this magnified view, isthmus of the cingulate gyrus can be well-visualized. The isthmus connects the cingulate gyrus with the parahippocampal gyrus.

Another hazard in this approach is injury to the splenium of the corpus callosum. This can result in a posterior disconnection syndrome. Patients would have a left visual hemianomia,

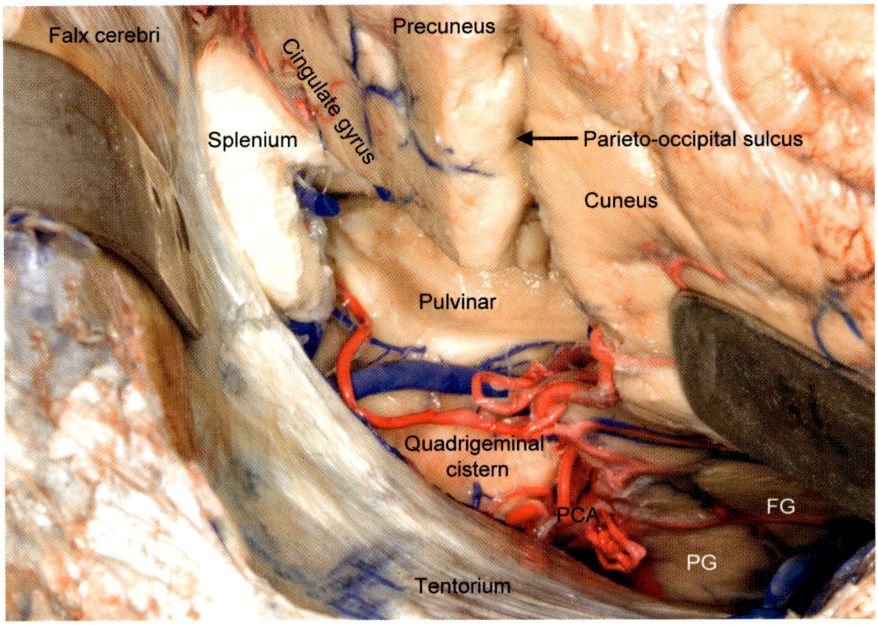

Fig. 6.8: After removal of the isthmus, the pulvinar thalamus is lateral and deep to the splenium. Deep and inferiorly, one can see a glimpse of the fusiform and the parahippocampal gyri.
(PG: Parahippocampal gyrus; FG: Fusiform gyrus; PCA: Posterior cerebral artery).

the inability to name stimuli presented in the left hemifield, if damage was posterior and dorsal corpus callosum. Left hemialexia, the inability to read words only in the left visual field, can occur, if damage was ventral and posterior along the corpus callosum.

Hydrocephalus, due to violating the ventricle while attempting gross total resection, can present as a postoperative complication, if hemostasis is not meticulously evaluated. In these instances, ½ × ½ patties are useful for plugging up the ventricle to prevent blood from tumor infiltrating through. If there is further concern, a ventriculostomy can be left in place and be weaned off postoperatively a few days later.

REFERENCES

1. Guillain GG. A case of tumor of the splenium of the corpus callosum. Ann de med. 1922;11:33.
2. Horrax G. Extirpation of a huge pinealoma from a patient with pubertas praecox. Arch Neurol Psychiatry. 1937;37:385-97.
3. Poppen JL. The right occipital approach to a pinealoma. J Neurosurg. 1966;25:706-10.
4. Poppen JL, Marino R. Pinealomas and tumors of the posterior portion of the third ventricle. J Neurosurg. 1968;28:357-64.
5. Jamieson KG. Excision of pineal tumors. J Neurosurg. 1971;35:550-3.
6. Malikovic A, Vucetic B, Milisavljevic M, Tosevski J, Sazdanovic P, Milojevic B, et al. Occipital sulci of the human brain: variability and morphometry. Anat Sci Int. 2012;87(2):61-70.
7. Flores LP. Occipital lobe morphological anatomy: anatomical and surgical aspects. Arq Neuropsiquiatr. 2002;60(3A):566-71.

8. Figueiredo EG, Beer-Furlan A, Welling LC, Ribas EC, Schafranski M, Crawford N, et al. Microsurgical approaches to the ambient cistern region: an anatomic and qualitative study. World Neurosurg. 2016;87:584-90.
9. Allen IM. A Clinical study of tumours involving the occipital lobe. Brain. 1930;53(2):194-243.
10. Jittapiromsak P, Deshmukh P, Nakaji P, Spetzler RF, Preul MC. Comparative analysis of posterior approaches to the medial temporal region: supracerebellar transtentorial versus occipital transtentorial. Neurosurgery. 2009;64(3):35-42.
11. Talacchi A, Hasabelliu A, Fasano T, Gerosa M. Interhemispheric approach to tumors of the posterior gyrus rectus. Clin Neurol Neurosurg. 2013;115(5):597-602.
12. Tseng KY, Lin JH, Lin EY, Ma HI. Occipital interhemispheric approach without excision of tentorium for the tumor in the medial temporal region: technical note. Surg Neurol. 2009;71(4):448-50.
13. Bassinouni H, Asgari S, Konig JH, Stolke D. Meningiomas of the falcotentorial junction: selection of the surgical approach according to the tumor type. Surg Neurol. 2008;69(4):339-49.
14. Chi JH, Lawton MT. Posterior interhemispheric approach: surgical technique, application to vascular lesions, and benefits of gravity retraction. Neurosurgery. 2006;59(1):41-9.
15. Terasaka S, Sawamura Y, Kamiyama H, Fukushima T. Surgical approaches for the treatment of aneurysms on the P2 segment of the posterior cerebral artery. Neurosurgery. 2000;47(2):359-6.
16. Tokunaga K, Tamiya T, Date I. Transient memory disturbance after removal of an intraventricular trigonal meningioma by a parieto-occipital interhemispheric precuneus approach: Case Report. Surg Neurol. 2006;65(2):167-9.
17. Winn HR, Youmans JR. Youman's Neurological Surgery. Philadelphia: Saunders; 2004.
18. Yaşargil MG. Microneurosurgery. Stuttgart: Thieme; 1996.

CHAPTER 7

Surgical Approaches and Strategies in Lesions of the Cingulate Gyrus

Richard W Byrne

INTRODUCTION

The cingulate gyrus represents the anterior superior extent of the limbic system. The cingulate gyrus can be thought of as a continuation of the parahippocampal gyrus. This relationship is most clear during embryological development. Between the 13th and 18th weeks of human development, the hippocampus recedes into the temporal lobe, leaving the indusium griseum as a gray matter remnant on top of the newly formed corpus callosum. Just superior to this lies the cingulate gyrus. The cingulate gyrus is bordered by the corpus callosum below, the cingulate sulcus above, the interhemispheric fissure medially and the descending white matter fibers laterally. Immediately above and adjacent to the cingulate sulcus from anterior to posterior is the septal area, the superior frontal gyrus, the paracentral lobule, and the superior parietal lobule.

SURGICAL APPROACHES

Natural approaches to the cingulate gyrus almost always involve an interhemispheric approach. An exception to this is in a case where the lesion reaches the cortex and provides a corridor to the cingulate pathology. Occasionally, the best approach to cingulate gyrus lesions is transfalcine from a contralateral hemisphere craniotomy. This is often the case for small lesions in which an ipsilateral exposure would not allow a safe trajectory, or in which large veins bridge the ipsilateral gap between the brain and the superior sagittal sinus. A careful study of the preoperative magnetic resonance imaging (MRI) will identify these cases. Other than this rare exception, most pathology is approached ipsilateral, intrahemispheric. In order to improve access, a lumbar drain or a lesion side down approach may be helpful.

Once the interhemispheric exposure is obtained, the large draining veins bridging the gap should be preserved. In order to aid this, minimal retraction, frequent irrigation, and covering with moistened gel foam is useful. Interhemispheric exposure is typically simple until the cingulate gyrus is reached. The two cingulate gyri are often adherent and sometimes interdigitating. The cingulate gyrus is sometimes misidentified as the corpus callosum to the uninitiated. The corpus callosum in surgical exposure is unmistakable once identified. It is usually useful to expose the corpus callosum in cingulate surgical cases in order to clearly identify the pericallosal arteries. They can then be protected, and can be followed anteriorly to the bifurcation of the pericallosal artery and the callosomarginal artery. The callosomarginal artery typically rises superiorly and enters or runs parallel to the cingulate sulcus. Preservation of the major branches of these arteries is essential to preservation of leg motor function. As such, early identification of these arteries is advised. In order to preserve these arteries when removing tumors in the cingulate gyrus a proximal to distal resection can be helpful, following the obtuse angles of the arteries, and avoiding the acute angles of arterial branching.

The final issue in removing cingulate lesions is deciding where the lateral resection should end. This is very clear in some well-demarcated lesions, but less clear in epilepsy surgery or in low-grade gliomas with a similar appearance and texture to gray matter. In cases below the paracentral lobule, subcortical electrical stimulation can be useful in a nonparalyzed patient. Somatosensory evoked potential (SSEP) and motor evoked potential (MEP) monitoring may also be used but may suffer from delay in warning of sensorimotor white matter disruption.

CASE 1: LEFT FRONTAL-CINGULATE GRADE II MIXED OLIO-ASTROCYTOMA; APPROACHED VIA LEFT FRONTAL INTERHEMISPHERIC CORRIDOR

History

A 29-year-old right-handed female with history of recent onset headache and confusion who presented with a generalized seizure. Magnetic resonance imaging (MRI) was consistent with a giant left frontal and cingulate mass displacing the entirety of the left frontal lobe, cingulate gyrus and frontal horn of the lateral ventricle (Fig. 7.1A). As such, a left frontal interhemispheric approach was planned.

Surgery

The patient was positioned supine and a bifrontal skin incision planned (Fig. 7.1B). A left frontal craniotomy was performed with the medial edge abutting the superior sagittal sinus. Dura was opened and reflected against the sinus. Subsequently, asleep motor mapping was performed to delineate the motor cortex posteriorly. Once confirmed, the resection ensued. The mass was approached by a combination of debulking and circumferential removal. The posterior and medial borders were defined by mapping and falx, respectively. Anterior and lateral borders of resection were guided by microscopic evaluation of tissue as well as neuronavigation. Resection planes continued until the ventricle was approached (Figs. 7.1C to H).

Postoperatively, the patient exhibited transient partial weakness on the right side which resolved fully by week 6 after the operation. Final pathology was consistent with mixed oligoastrocytoma grade II (Figs. 7.1I to L).

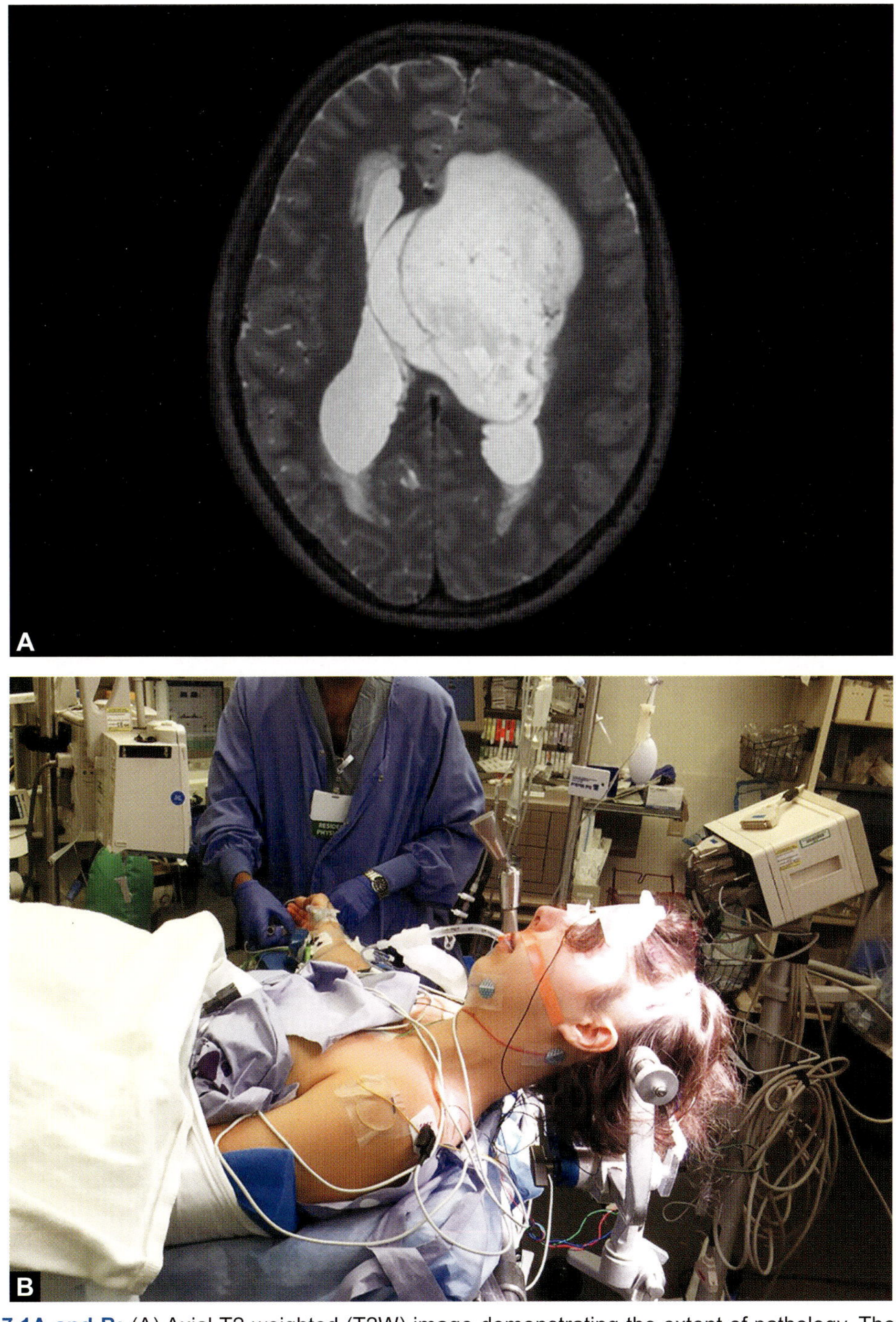

Figs. 7.1A and B: (A) Axial T2-weighted (T2W) image demonstrating the extent of pathology. The tumor is noted to involve the subcortical left frontal lobe with extension into the ventricular system. (B) Patient is positioned supine and head is fixated. A bifrontal skin incision is marked.

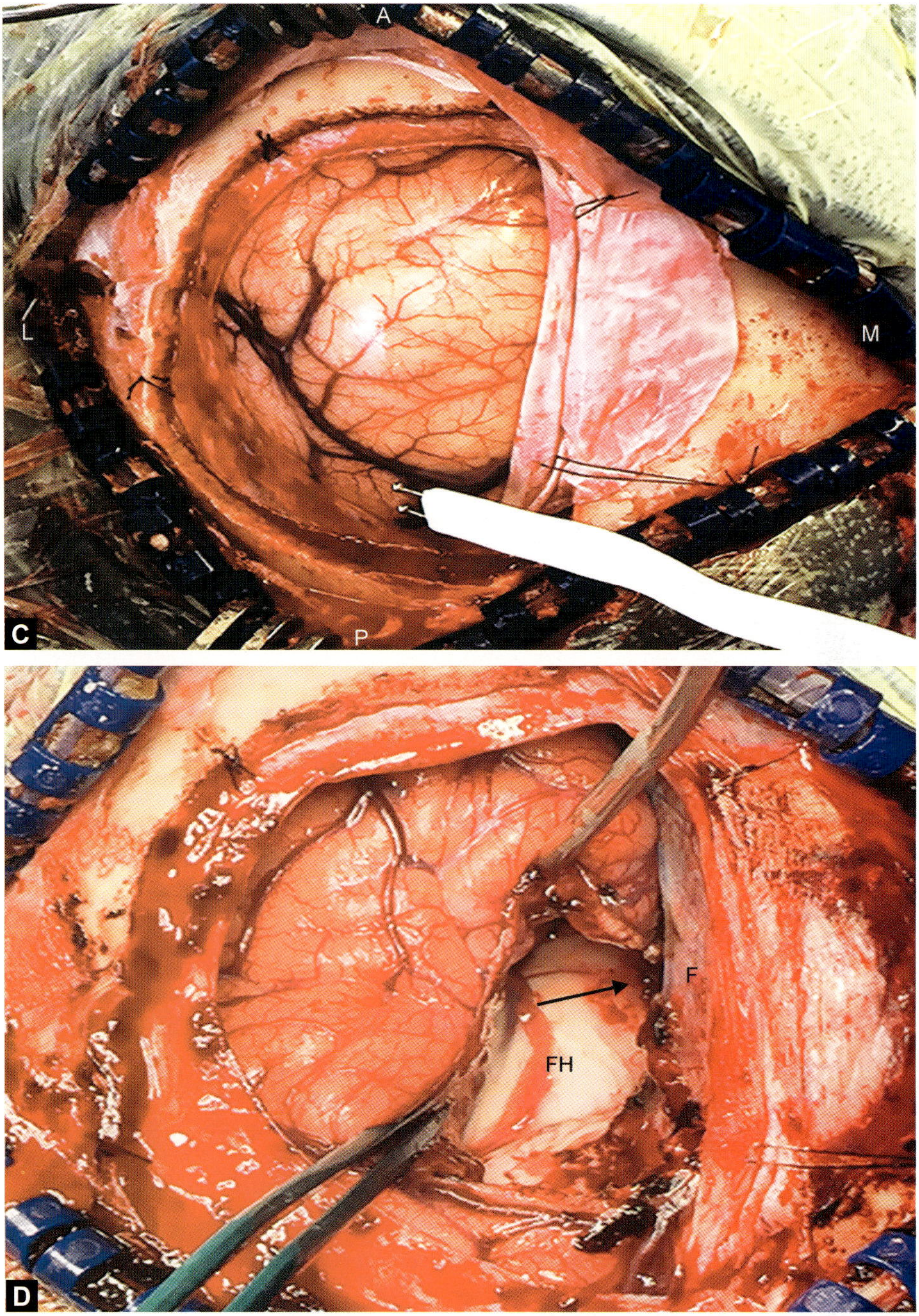

Figs. 7.1C and D: Intraoperative images: (C) Cortical mapping of the precentral gyrus. The visualized vein corresponds to the precentral sulcus and posterior margin of resection. (D) Resection cavity after removal of the tumor. Retraction of brain reveals contents of the left frontal horn (FH). The septum has been removed. Foramen of Monro (arrow) is visible (F: Falx; A: Anterior; P: Posterior; L: Lateral; M: Medial).

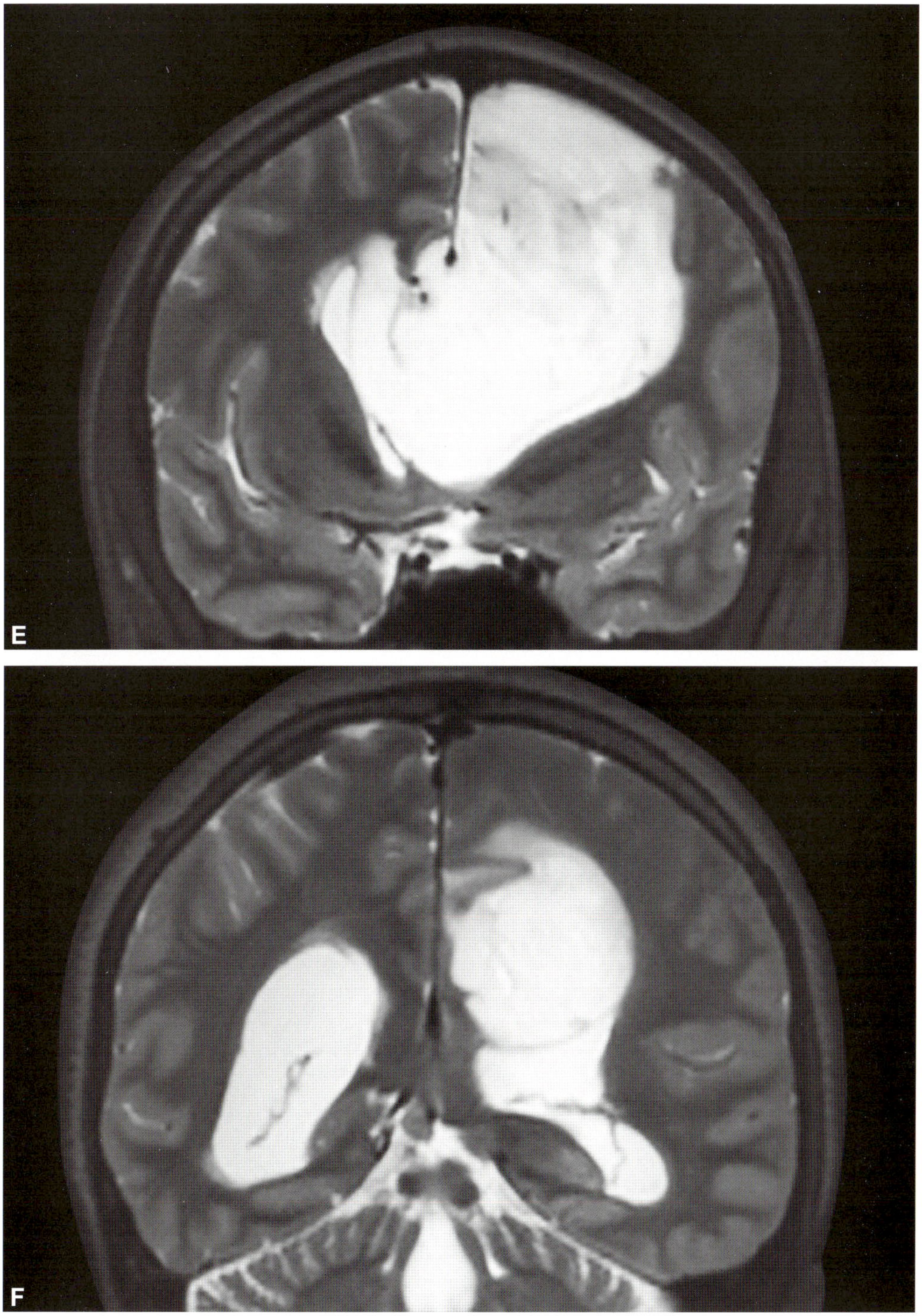

Figs. 7.1E and F

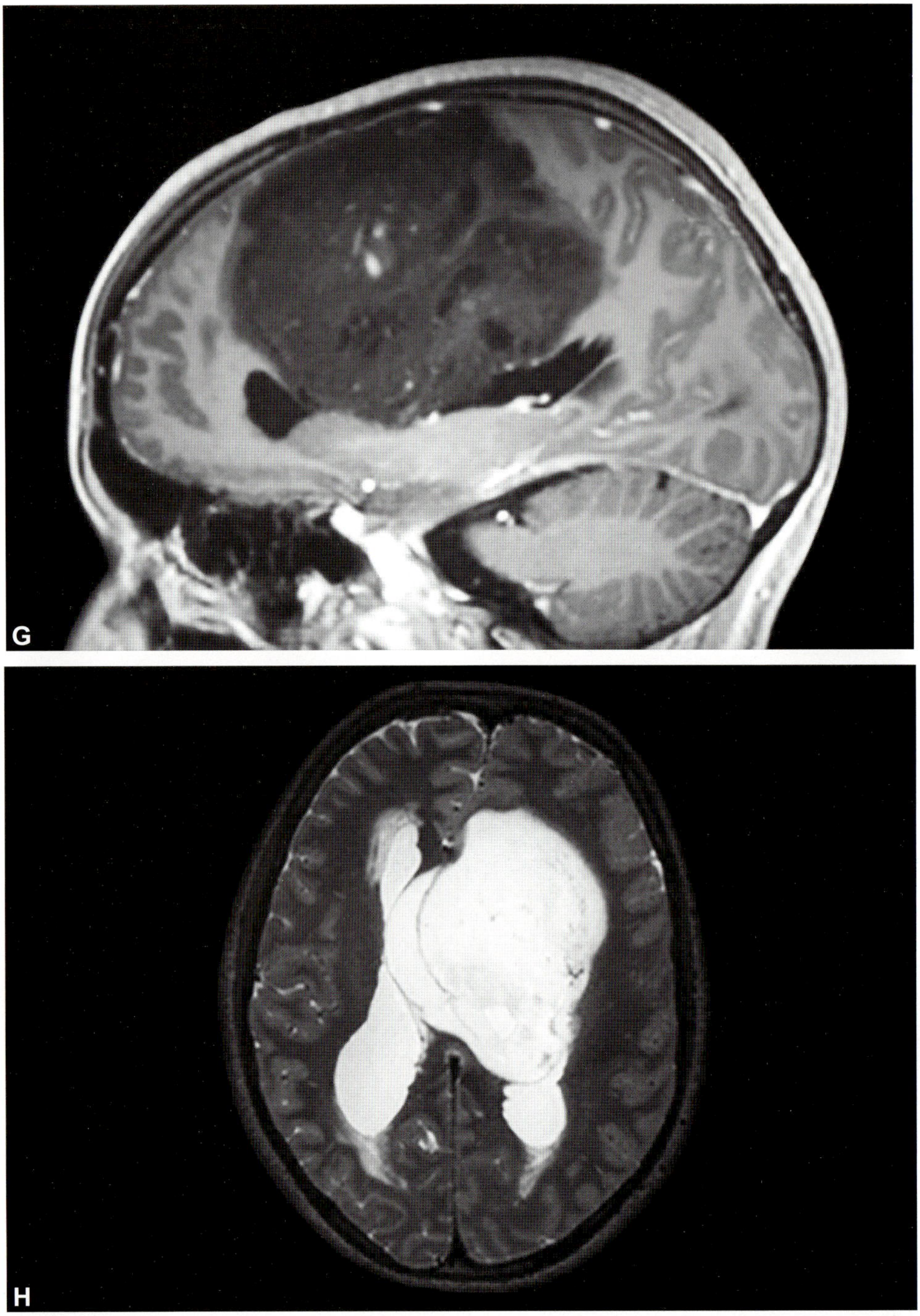

Figs. 7.1G and H

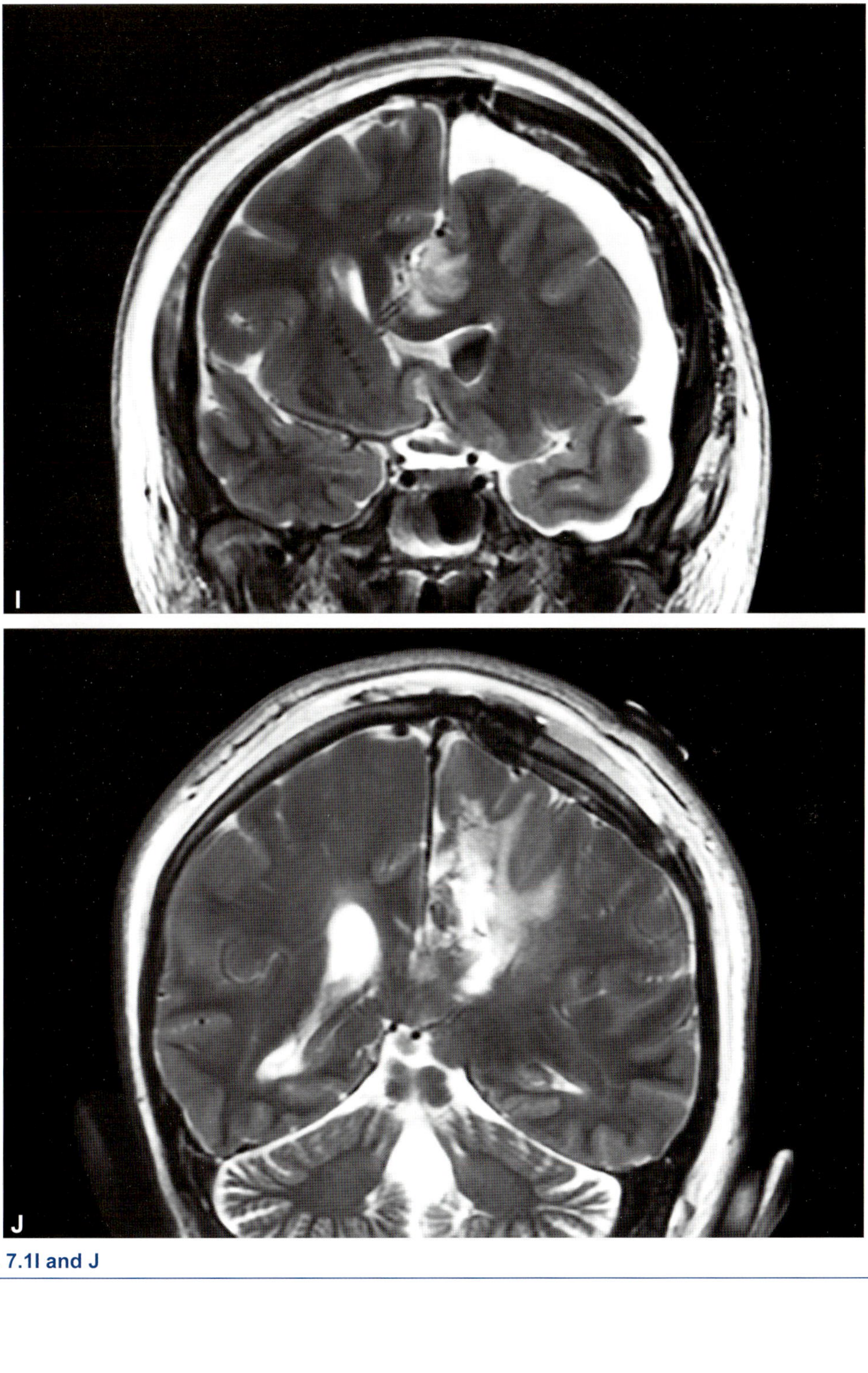

Figs. 7.1I and J

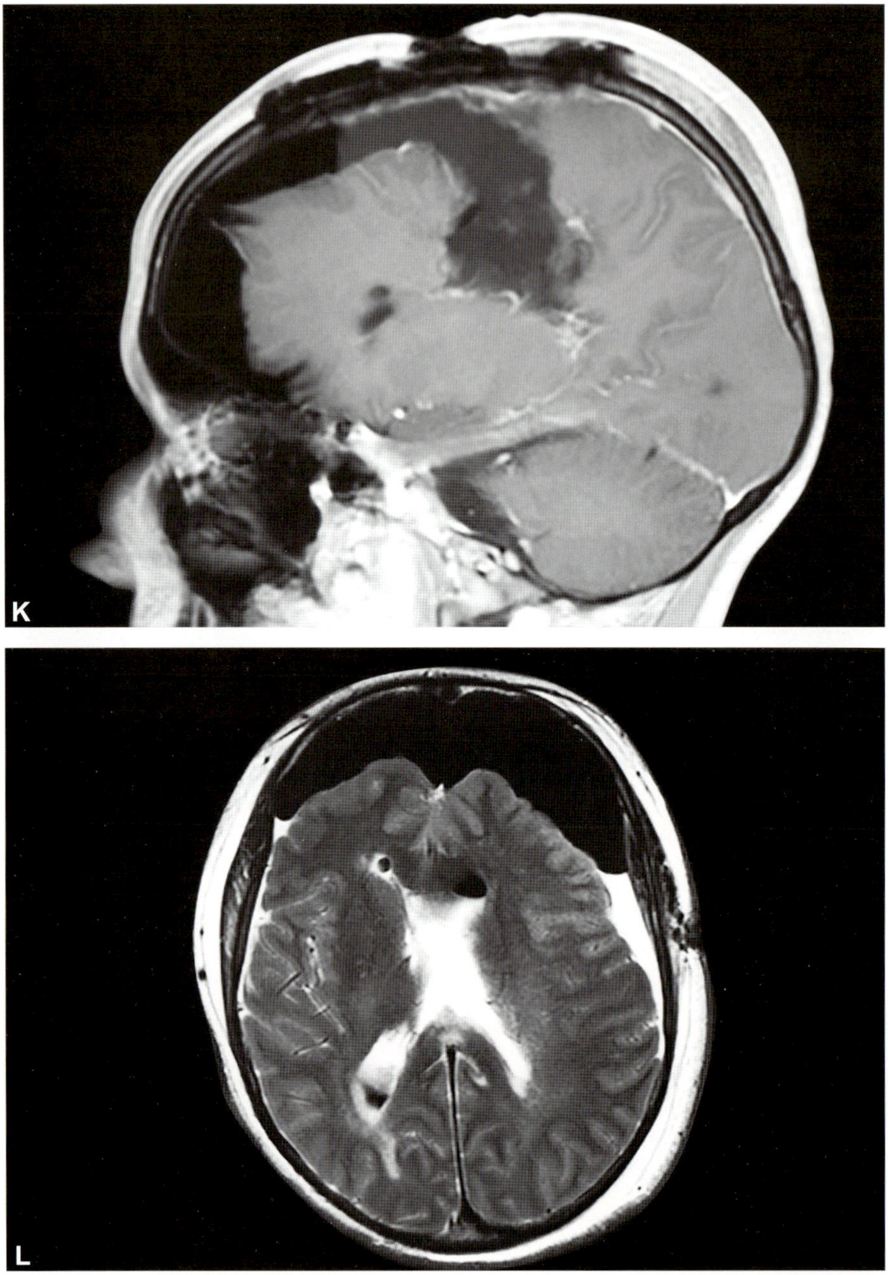

Figs. 7.1E to L: (E to H) Preoperative MRI images. (E and F) Coronal T2W images; (G) Sagittal T1 postcontrast image; (H) Axial T2W images. (I to L) Postoperative MRI images of the preoperative sequences demonstrating gross total resection.

CHAPTER

8

Brain Mapping during Surgery of the Limbic System

Sepehr Sani, Carter S Gerard, Richard W Byrne

INTRODUCTION

While concrete knowledge of classical anatomic descriptions of cortical language and motor locations are mandatory for each neurosurgeon, it is not sufficient for localizing eloquent cortices. Even in the normal brain, language function localization can be highly variable.[1-4] The inconstant location of eloquent cortex can present unique challenges to both tumor resection and surgical management of epileptic foci involving the limbic system. Tumors and/or epileptic foci within the limbic system may involve, invade or displace eloquent cortex. Cortical stimulation can reliably identify motor cortex in the anesthetized patient, while identification of language cortex requires an awake and cooperative subject. Intraoperative cortical stimulation mapping was first described over 80 years ago,[5] it remains the gold standard for in vivo identification of eloquent cortex allowing the neurosurgeon to maximize resection while minimizing risk to the patient.[6,7] In this chapter, we will focus on the techniques for cortical mapping and surgical treatment of pathology involving the limbic system and overlying eloquent cortex.

INDICATIONS

We define topographic regions of the brain with presumed eloquence similar to previously published studies,[8-14] which include the primary sensorimotor cortex of the pre- and post-central gyri, Wernicke's area (posterior portion of the superior temporal gyrus and the inferior parietal lobule), Broca's area (inferior posterior dominant frontal lobe), the calcarine visual cortex, the basal ganglia, internal capsule, thalamus and the white matter paths of each. If any part of the lesion is found to infiltrate these regions it is regarded as being located in presumed eloquent brain; if it approaches, but does not clearly involve these regions it is considered near eloquent and if it is situated in a separate anatomic location it is considered noneloquent.

While lesions distant from eloquent anatomic structures do not require further pre-operative functional investigation, it is prudent to consider preoperative functional imaging in lesions involving eloquent and near eloquent brain to help define the critical structures within the proposed operative field. Patients with pathology within the areas considered to be eloquent or near eloquent cortex may benefit from intraoperative cortical stimulation. If language mapping is required a patient must be without major dysphasia or confusion, and have the ability to tolerate an awake craniotomy.

INTEGRATING WITH FUNCTIONAL IMAGING

While the use of functional magnetic resonance imaging (fMRI) allows the surgeon to better assess the relationship of a lesion to eloquent cortex, there are considerable limitation, especially when mapping language areas. Several recent studies have shown relatively reliable motor cortex mapping when compared to intraoperative stimulation.[1,11,15,16] However, while fMRI has largely replaced Wada test for language lateralization, fMRI does not allow for precise localization of language which is reflected by the wide range of reported results in the literature. A review of five studies showed language mapping sensitivity from 59 to 100% and specificity from 0 to 97% when compared to intraoperative stimulation.[11,17] Various authors have used newer noninvasive technologies for anatomic mapping such magnetoencephalography (MEG) and transcranial magnetic stimulation (TMS).[18-21] Advanced preoperative functional imaging may serve two important purposes:

1. Neuroplasticity may induce migration of functional activity to other neighboring regions in cortical dysplasia or tumor infiltrated brain, which is why minimal or no neurological deficits are seen in some patients with slow growing low-grade gliomas. Thus, a better understanding of the true functional eloquence of the anatomically eloquent region under investigation is gained. This finding has redefined the term "eloquence" and indeed resulted in a greater number of successful resections that were previously considered as being part of anatomically eloquent cortex.
2. It enables the surgeon to understand the most dangerous regions of the epileptic foci or tumor with regard to neurological morbidity and estimate the extent of safe resection prior to the operation.[22-24] This can aid discussions with the patient and multidisciplinary care-providers considering adjuvant and neoadjuvant treatment options.

PREOPERATIVE PREPARATION

The Patient

In preparation for surgery, a thorough understanding of the patient's baseline neurocognitive status is needed. We consider formal neuropsychological evaluation of patients with lesions involving or near the speech cortex. Often there are "silent" deficits present preoperatively that may go unnoticed.[25] Furthermore, identification of cognitive deficits may guide the resection approach and extent irrespective of pure motor or language findings in addition to monitoring postoperative recovery.[26]

The cornerstone of a successful cortical mapping assisted resection is patient cooperation in the awake setting. This is particularly important in language mapping. During the preoperative clinic visit, a detailed rehearsal and review of expectations during the awake portion of the operation can be very helpful in allaying patient anxiety and ensuring a cooperative patient.

If language mapping is anticipated, preoperatively the patient is extensively counseled on the nature of intraoperative testing and undergoes a baseline language evaluation as follows: the patient is asked to count from 1 to 50, name objects seen on a computer generated slide show, read single words projected on a computer screen sequentially, repeat complex sentences, and write words and sentences on paper. Language deficits are classified as anomia when the patient is unable to name an object but able to repeat sentences and has fluent speech. Alexia is defined as retention of the ability to write spell, but with reading errors. Aphasia may be expressive, receptive, or mixed. Mild language errors such as paraphasic errors are not considered in resection planning. Patient should have 80% language comprehension preoperatively in order to be considered for awake speech mapping.

Equipment

The following is a listing of the standard material and equipment used at the senior author's institution for cortical and subcortical brain mapping during resection operation:

- Image guidance for anatomical localization and verification.
- Electroencephalographic (EEG) monitoring of cortical surface by placement of an electrode strip or grid on the cortical surface to monitor after-discharges during stimulation.
- Appropriate EEG cables and strips or grids. One to two six contact strips are placed adjacent to the stimulated area.
- Cortical stimulation probe and box with power source verified [e.g. Ojemann Cortical Stimulator (Radionics Corp., Burlington, MA) or another commercially available probe].
- Counted and linked map tags for cortical identification during mapping.
- Cold saline or Ringer's solution for irrigation to abrogate an induced seizure during stimulation.
- Neuropsychological assessment team with naming cards for speech mapping.
- Dedicated and experienced neuroanesthesiologist.

Anesthetic Considerations

For general anesthesia, a routine cranial neuroanesthesia protocol is followed. Pharmacological paralysis and high concentrations of inhalation anesthetic agents are avoided. In awake craniotomy cases, the following regimen is employed: Before incision, midazolam (2 mg; avoided, if EEG to be recorded) and fentanyl (50–100 mg) are administered. During surgery, either propofol (50–100 mcg/kg of body weight per minute; avoided, if EEG will be recorded) or dexmedetomidine (0.2–0.7 mcg/kg/hr) and remifentanil (0.05–0.2 mcg/kg/min) are given. Local anesthesia is given along the Mayfield pin sites as well as a circumferential scalp field block. A mixture of 0.5% lidocaine, 0.25% Marcaine (bupivacaine hydrochloride), and epinephrine (1/200,000) are used. Once the craniotomy is performed, intradural injections along either side of the middle meningeal artery are given in cases involving the middle fossa. Anesthetic agents are discontinued at this time until mapping is completed. Painful portions of the operation, such as early portions of the exposure and dural opening are managed by sedation, patient reassurance and transient increase in propofol infusion rate. In cases of insufficient sedation, supplementary boluses of propofol (0.5 mg/kg) are given and the infusion rate may be increased to 125 mg/kg/min. Nausea or vomiting can be controlled with intravenous droperidol (1.2–2.5 mg) or metoclopramide (5–10 mg). The patient is asked to hyperventilate before dural opening. Once mapping is complete, sedatives are restarted. Intraoperative seizures due to cortical stimulation have been reported in up to 24% of cases.[27,28] Epilepsy patients are at particularly increased risk of intraoperative seizures due to decreased anticonvulsant levels. These seizures, whether focal or general, are usually transient and can be suppressed by application of local ice-cold Ringer's solution and a bolus of intravenous propofol (1 mg/kg).[12] If airway control is of concern, tracheal intubation may be necessary.

Preparations and Positioning

Patient comfort is paramount in cortical mapping operations. Often during longer operations in an awake patient, hip or neck pain can cause more discomfort than the actual surgery. Extra padding of all pressure points is essential. The neck position should look comfortable. Side positioners should be placed on both sides along with safety straps and the patient should be securely taped to the bed. Wrists should be secured with restraints. The drapes need to be elevated to allow direct visualization for seizures, airway concerns, testing such as object naming, and to avoid claustrophobia.

After positioning, monitors are attached, an indwelling urinary catheter is inserted, and oxygen delivery via nasal cannula is provided. Usually the semilateral position is preferred using a padded roll for back support. The semisitting position may be needed for some cases involving motor or sensory cortex. Medications such as mannitol and dexamethasone, as well as antibiotics are given prior to making the incision.

Craniotomy Considerations

The draping is performed accordingly to allow the anesthesiologist and examiner the full view of the patients face as well as contralateral arm and leg for intraoperative monitoring of the patient's neurologic and respiratory status. A localized craniotomy is performed using standard neurosurgical technique with the assistance of neuronavigation. A tailored craniotomy is preferred, including the underlying lesion or seizure focus, along with exposure of surrounding areas. The patient remains under heavy sedation until the craniotomy is complete. Ideally, the patient awakes as the dura is opened. Pain upon awakening can be addressed with local anesthetic. Often pain is related to the temporalis muscle which is difficult to block. Releasing traction on the muscle can relieve pain.

In case of a posterior temporal-parietal-occipital focus, a generous craniotomy is preferred with exposure of the occipital, occipital-parietal and posterior temporal language areas for testing. After the durotomy, neuronavigation is used to identify the cortical margins of the lesion. Expected locations of central sulcus and sylvian fissure are also identified. All margins and landmarks are labeled on the cortical surface.

Stimulation Mapping

Somatosensory Evoked Potential Recordings

Evoked potential recording can be used to localize the central sulcus.[29,30] This is particularly helpful in cases in which underlying lesions have distorted normal anatomy. The technique is performed by placing an electrode strip perpendicular across the proposed location of central sulcus. A contralateral suprathreshold median nerve stimulation is made, an N20 wave is recorded over the hand somatosensory cortex, and a phase reversal is observed across the fissure. This process is performed several times as the strip is moved along the sensorimotor cortex. Recording is usually begun 3–4 cm above the sylvian fissure. Two or three recordings are usually needed to localize the central sulcus. The hand region is the most readily identifiable area and is generally localized to 4–6 cm above the sylvian fissure. Once identified, the sulcus is labeled accordingly and the strip is removed. Continuous somatosensory evoked potential (SSEP) or motor evoked response can be continued through the operation. Evoked potential recording can be performed in the awake patient or under general anesthesia.

Electrocorticography

In patients with intractable epilepsy, electrocorticography (ECoG) may be used in order to identify the abnormal interictal spikes. The technique requires the presence of a neurophysiologist or epileptologist with neurophysiology expertise in the operating room for recording interpretation. An electrode grid is laid over the cortical area of interest and several minutes of electrocortical activity are recorded. Areas with abnormal interictal spikes are marked.[31] Surgical resection of these areas depends on their functional importance based on motor or language mapping. ECoG is also employed in monitoring of after-discharges during sensorimotor or language mapping as described in the succeeding section.

Sensorimotor Stimulation

Cortical mapping begins with a function check by stimulating the temporalis muscle, if exposed, and confirming visual contraction. If no contraction is seen up to 10 mA of stimulation, a systemic check is done (cable connections, paralytic levels, stimulation parameters, battery, etc.) It is important to remember that the bipolar stimulators are designed to be used in only 5–10 cases and are then replaced in order to avoid potential disconnection. The localization of pre- and postcentral gyri is confirmed by direct cortical stimulation after identification with evoked potentials. Detailed somatotopic mapping is also possible with cortical stimulation. This technique is used when the lesion or seizure focus is close to or involves sensorimotor locations. Stimulation is performed using an Ojemann Cortical Stimulator (Radionics Corp., Burlington, MA). Primary sensory cortex is mapped with the patient awake. Stimulation parameters of 1–2 mA total, with a frequency of 60 Hz and a pulse duration of 1 ms are used. Cortical patches of 1 cm^3 are stimulated sequentially with rest periods between stimulations. The probe is applied to the cortex for 3 sec duration and the patient is asked to report the onset and location of any perceived paresthesias. Stimulation starts in the suprasylvian portion of the sensory gyrus and advanced superiorly, thereby sequentially identifying the tongue, lip, and hand sensory areas.

If the operation is being performed under general anesthesia, only motor mapping is possible.[34] Stimulation parameters remain the same, but usually a higher threshold of initial stimulation is used (3 mA). Stimulation intensity increases until contralateral movement is observed by the anesthesiologist or the examiner. Amplitudes greater than 14 mA are not recommended in motor cortex stimulation. Congruent with sensory mapping, stimulation is initiated in the suprasylvian region in 1 cm^3 patches and moves superiorly along the gyrus until somatotopic mapping of tongue, lips, thumb, hand, and arm are obtained sequentially. If mapping of motor leg region is needed, stimulation is given through a strip electrode that is inserted in the interhemispheric fissure. Seizures, focal and general, can occur during motor mapping and have been reported in up to 24% of cases.[27,28] They are usually transient. Application of ice cold Ringer's solution for 5–10 sec is often effective at breaking the seizures. A bolus of intravenous propofol (1 mg/kg)[12] can also be given as adjunct to stop the seizure. Areas stimulated are labeled by the linked map tags that are connected to the surgical drapes. A picture may be taken at the end of mapping and the tags are removed.

Language Mapping

Language mapping is done in the awake patient when the lesion involves the dominant perisylvian frontotemporal region. Preoperative language evaluation and counseling has been described earlier in this chapter. Intraoperative language mapping is not useful in patients with significant language deficits. Intraoperatively, Broca's area is identified by stimulation induced speech arrest. Mapping is initiated at stimulation parameters of 1.5–3 mA, frequency of 50–60 Hz, and pulse duration of 1 ms. Once identified, cortical patches of 5 mm are stimulated sequentially with rest periods between stimulations. The probe is applied to the cortex for 1–3 sec and the patient is monitored. Each cortical patch is tested up to three times. Electrocorticography is monitored to determine the threshold for after-discharges. It is important to keep all stimulation below this threshold and meticulously monitor for after-discharges as they can produce false localizing results during mapping and may lead to a clinical seizure. For each site, the patient is tested for counting errors, object naming errors, and word reading errors as they are presented on naming cards. A cortical area is considered positive for language function if the patient is unable to count, name objects, repeat words or read words in two out of three stimulations.[32] Positive sites are labeled by sterile labels on the cortex (Figs. 8.1A to F) and marked using neuronavigation. It is also important to move to a different area of the cortex after completing stimulation in order to prevent summation and subsequent seizure activity. Usually no more than 25–30 sites are tested around the intended resection site to delineate the positive language areas. All positive language areas, vascular supplies, and white matter connections must be preserved during resection with a margin of 1 cm.[4,33-35] In anterior temporal resections of the dominant hemisphere, resections within 2 cm of a positive language area, particularly stimulation-induced anomia, will produce a mild but identifiable general language deficit observed on an aphasia battery administered 1 month after the operation.[36]

If all tested areas are negative for language errors and the mapping team is confident in the equipment and technique (stimulating upto after-discharge), wider cortical exposure is not necessary and the resection can be carried out based on delineated margins of the lesion or seizure focus. The cortical incision is made in a "silent" area first and resection is carried out.

Subcortical stimulation may be performed to preserve essential fibers. This typically requires higher levels of stimulation. Once mapping is completed, additional anesthetic agent may be given for patient comfort. It may be difficult to distinguish the mechanism of speech

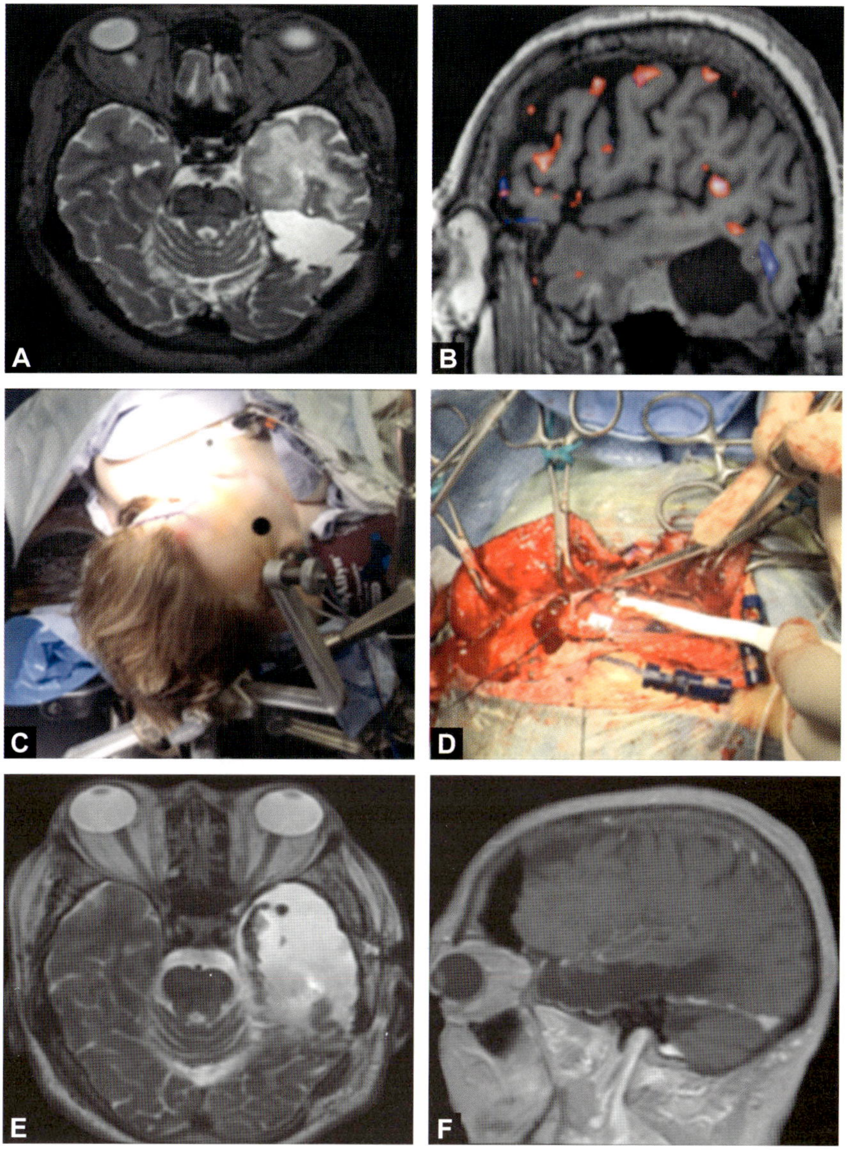

Figs. 8.1A to F: (A) A 63-year-old female with a history of left temporal anaplastic oligodendroglioma with 1p/19q deletions s/p resection 10 years earlier presents for evaluation due to radiographic progression on serial imaging. (B) Functional MRI showed bilateral speech with activity at the superior posterior border of the existing resection cavity. (C) The patient was taken to the operating room for awake craniotomy for speech mapping. (D) Intraoperative speech mapping produced arrest during inferior parietal stimulation. (E and F) The surgery was completed without development of deficits. Postoperative imaging showed a gross total resection despite dominant temporal involvement.

arrest during stimulation of the inferior prefrontal cortex as this area is intimately involved in both language and motor function. Speech arrest can be attributed to a stimulus disturbance of language function or arrest of motor activity. Indeed a combined language and motor function in these cortical areas has been suggested.[13,37] These areas, when encountered, should be marked as eloquent cortex and preserved, as their resection will lead to postoperative language deficits.

Stimulation Pitfalls

Although identification of the eloquent areas of cortex by stimulation mapping is considered the gold standard, this technique is not without limitations. Indeed a positive cortical finding during stimulation may reflect retrograde activation of another area through network activity. Another issue is that an area is found to be positive by stimulation may be redundantly represented (whether as a function of the original network or due to plasticity secondary to the underlying) and hence amenable to resection.

Another issue worthy of mention is negative mapping. This technique has been reported as an alternative to positive mapping with the advantage of a more limited craniotomy, exposure, and operative time.[14,38-40] This technique is of great value for the experienced practitioner. However, the caveat lies in the potential for false negative findings in less experienced centers. Technical issues, suboptimal patient cooperation, or insufficient levels of stimulation can skew negative mapping results and result in resection of potentially eloquent areas. Furthermore, in operations involving seizure foci or lesions (such as low-grade glioma) that do not have visible anatomical borders, the extent of resection is defined by the borders of positive mapping, not negative mapping. In most cases, however, negative mapping is adequate for safe resection in and around eloquent centers.

Subcortical Stimulation Mapping

Once resection continues past the cortical surface, it is possible and sometimes necessary to continue stimulation mapping. Subcortical stimulation mapping (SSM) refers to stimulating the descending (or ascending in case of primary sensory cortex) white matter network tracks that connect various cortical structures to each other to deep nuclei as well as stimulation of the basal ganglia or thalamic areas. The technique is the same as cortical mapping but stimulation parameters are generally higher than cortical mapping. The resection is carried out incrementally using anatomic landmarks and neuronavigation, with frequent confirmation by SSM before proceeding to the next area. It should be emphasized that subcortical white matter tracks are as eloquent as the cortical structures. Preservation of theses essential tracks is especially challenging due to the poorly defined borders of subcortical anatomy and the tendency of adjacent pathology to distort the expected trajectory of the white matter.

Surgical Endpoints

The goal of stimulation mapping is to allow the surgeon maximal extent of resection with preservation of neurological function. Upon completion of mapping, resection starts from the least eloquent area and proceed to the most eloquent area. In the awake patient, continued motor and speech assessment will alert the surgeon to any new deficits. These assessments should increase in frequency as needed as the operation proceeds toward mapped eloquent areas.

Resection involving motor cortex or subcortical areas should stop at least 5 mm from identified eloquent areas.[41] Resection can be continued to the pre- or postcentral sulcus, if there are clearly identified and white matter is spared. Low-grade gliomas often respect gyri. The tumor can expand gyri, pushing into presumed functional areas without infiltrating. They appear to occupy eloquent regions, while in reality only displacing them, and can then be identified by counting the gyri. It has been the senior author's experience that stopping the resection when the patient's motor examination is 3/5 or mild dysphasia will result is an intact patient at 6 weeks follow-up unless there is a vascular injury or descending white matter has been interrupted.

Alternatively for continuous motor mapping, a six-contact strip can be placed on the precentral gyrus for continuous motor stimulation mapping. Continuous, repeated assessment of an awake patient while operating in or near eloquent cortex remains the safest way to maximize resection and preserve function. When operating around language areas, resection should stop 1 cm from any identified speech area or if there is any change in language testing.

EPILEPSY SPECIFIC TECHNIQUES IN ELOQUENT CORTEX

Multiple Subpial Transections

Multiple subpial transection (MST) is a surgical technique used to disrupt synchrony of seizure foci by disputing horizontal oriented fibers, while minimizing functional disruption of afferent and efferent fibers, which run vertical.[17,27,28] At the same time, seizures in part spread horizontally through the gray matter. The goal of this surgery is to inhibit synchronization and spread of the seizure focus while minimizing damage to the cortex. The first large series of MST was reported 1989,[26] the technique can be used in eloquent cortex when permanent deficits are not acceptable. MST may be used to treat patients with epileptogenic lesions of the speech, motor, or primary sensory cortex.

Multiple subpial transection may be performed under general anesthesia following extraoperative subdural grid mapping or awake if intraoperative language mapping is planned. A standard craniotomy is performed to ensure adequate exposure for functional mapping and ECoG. If subsequent testing reveals the seizure focus to reside in eloquent and noneloquent cortex, surgical resection may be performed in the noneloquent cortex to within 1 cm of language cortex and to the border of sensory and motor cortex.[20,29] White matter pathways and vascular supplies are preserved. If repeat ECoG does not show significant resolution of the interictal activity or if the primary residual focus lies within eloquent cortex, MST may be performed at the apex of the implicated gyri. Transections are made in the direction perpendicular to the long axis of the gyrus. If resolution of the seizure focus is seen with ECoG, no additional transection is performed.

A pliable wire that is bent into a 4 mm blunt hook is used to carry out the transection. The hook of the subpial transector (Whisler-Morrell Subpial Transector, Redman Neurotechnologists, Lake Zurich, IL) measures 4 mm, the average depth of gray matter in the neocortex.[28] Prior to transection, the gyral and microgyral patterns are closely inspected. The surrounding and bypassing vessels are defined. Once ECoG has been performed, the transections are started at the apex of the targeted gyrus in order to avoid interference from subsequent subarachnoid bleeding. The transection is begun by opening a hole the pia at the edge of a sulcus with a 20-gauge needle. The transector enters the gray matter through this opening, and then is advanced in a straight line across the vertex of the gyrus in a direction perpendicular to the long axis of the gyrus. The hook is then withdrawn along the same path, with the tip of the hook visible just below the pia.[25,42,43] The next transection line is made parallel to and 5 mm from the first. Great care must be taken to note the course of the major blood vessels, particularly around the sylvian and interhemispheric fissures. When transections must be performed in the depths of a sulcus or fissure, the hook is inserted upside down, with the tip pointed away from the pial surface. This lessens the likelihood of damaging a vessel in the sulcus or fissure. The obtuse angle of the hook also helps lessen the likelihood of injury to vessels. In cases of perisylvian-onset epilepsy, it is often useful to open the sylvian fissure to record from the depths of the fissure and transect under direct vision. In some cases, transection at 5 mm intervals is not possible because of microgyral patterns or a large confluence of vessels that may cover the area to be transected.

During the early postoperative period, most patients who undergo MST in eloquent cortex have subtle, transient deficits corresponding to the area transected. These deficits are most evident in the first week after surgery. As the edema and microhemorrhages resolve, most patients return to their baseline function within 6 weeks.[24]

The results of MST in the literature must be separated into cases of MST alone and MST with concomitant resection. Spencer et al. performed a meta-analysis on 212 patients who underwent MST at six epilepsy centers.[37] In cases of MST alone without resection, they reported rates of excellent outcome with regard to seizure control of 71% for generalized epilepsy, 62% for complex partial epilepsy, and 63% for simple partial seizures. However, it is more common to use a combination of MST and resection as seen in the series of Morrell and Whisler,[26] as it is rare for a seizure focus to lie entirely in eloquent cortex. A total of 82% of patients in this category were seizure free or had a significant reduction in their seizures (Engel's class I to III) Although the majority of patients exhibited worthwhile improvement, the initial report by Morrell of 52% being free of seizures was not sustained later in the series.[26] The meta-analysis reported by Spencer and coauthors showed similar results for patients who underwent resection with MST. The patients had marked seizure reduction (>95% reduction) reported in 87% of patients with generalized seizures, 68% of patients with complex partial seizures, and 68% of patients with simple partial epilepsy.[37] However, long-term results are not as favorable in other series, with 18.5% seizure recurrence rate with 5 years of follow-up.[32,36] This phenomenon has also been described in patients who have undergone resective epilepsy surgery.

Responsive Neurostimulation System

When a nonlesional seizure focus is located entirely in eloquent cortex, MST or a stimulation procedure, such as vagus nerve stimulation (VNS) or responsive neurostimulation system (RNS), are the only surgical options.[16,44,45] Currently, the only commercially available RNS is NeuroPace (NeuroPace, Mountain View, CA, USA). NeuroPace is a closed looped system that is designed to detect and interrupted electrical activity at the seizure focus at onset. The NeuroPace system was approved by the US Food and Drug Administration (FDA) as an adjunctive therapy for treatment of seizures in adult patients with partial onset seizures, who have no more than two epileptogenic foci, are refractory to more than or equal to two antiepileptic medications, and currently have frequent and disabling seizures.[41] The system includes one or two either depth and/or cortical electrodes/strips that can be used for recording and stimulation, along with a neurostimulator that is implanted in the skull. No cortical resection is performed, thus eliminating neurological deficit associated resection in the eloquent areas.

The use of RNS before MST enables long-term recording and improved foci localization. In our center, we consider RNS prior to performing MST when the seizure focus lies within eloquent cortex. However, other surgeons have argued that MST should be performed prior to RNS in order to avoid damage to underlying cortex caused by removal of adherent electrodes.

REFERENCES

1. Arora J, Pugh K, Westerveld M, Spencer S, Spencer DD, Todd Constable R. Language lateralization in epilepsy patients: fMRI validated with the Wada procedure. Epilepsia. 2009;50:2225-41.
2. Bizzi A, Blasi V, Falini A, Ferroli P, Cadioli M, Danesi U, et al. Presurgical functional MR imaging of language and motor functions: validation with intraoperative electrocortical mapping. Radiology. 2008;248:579-89.
3. Bowyer SM, Moran JE, Weiland BJ, Mason KM, Greenwald ML, Smith BJ, et al. Language laterality determined by MEG mapping with MR-FOCUSS. Epilepsy Behav EB. 2005;6:235-41.
4. Roux F-E, Boulanouar K, Lotterie J-A, Mejdoubi M, LeSage JP, Berry I. Language functional magnetic resonance imaging in preoperative assessment of language areas: correlation with direct cortical stimulation. Neurosurgery. 2003;52:1335-45; discussion 1345-47.
5. Szelényi A, Bello L, Duffau H, Fava E, Feigl GC, Galanda M, et al. Intraoperative electrical stimulation in awake craniotomy: methodological aspects of current practice. Neurosurg Focus. 2010;28:E7.
6. De Witt Hamer PC, Robles SG, Zwinderman AH, Duffau H, Berger MS. Impact of intraoperative stimulation brain mapping on glioma surgery outcome: a meta-analysis. J Clin Oncol. 2012;30:2559-65.
7. Duffau H, Capelle L, Denvil D, Sichez N, Gatignol P, Taillandier L, et al. Usefulness of intraoperative electrical subcortical mapping during surgery for low-grade gliomas located within eloquent brain regions: functional results in a consecutive series of 103 patients. J Neurosurg. 2003;98:764-78.
8. Berger MS. Lesions in functional ("eloquent") cortex and subcortical white matter. Clin Neurosurg. 1994;41:444-63.
9. Chang EF, Clark A, Smith JS, Polley M-Y, Chang SM, Barbaro NM, et al. Functional mapping-guided resection of low-grade gliomas in eloquent areas of the brain: improvement of long-term survival: clinical article. J Neurosurg. 2011;114:566-73.
10. Delev D, Send K, Wagner J, von Lehe M, Ormond DR, Schramm J, et al. Epilepsy surgery of the rolandic and immediate perirolandic cortex: surgical outcome and prognostic factors. Epilepsia. 2014;55:1585-93.
11. Kim SS, McCutcheon IE, Suki D, Weinberg JS, Ferson D, Heimberger AB, et al. Awake craniotomy for brain tumors near eloquent cortex: correlation of intraoperative cortical mapping with neurological outcomes in 309 consecutive patients. Neurosurgery. 2009;64:836-45.
12. Ojemann G. Awake operations with mapping in epilepsy. In: Schmidek HH, Sweet WH, (Eds). Operative Neurosurgical Techniques, 3rd edition. Philadelphia: WB Saunders; 1995. pp. 1317-22.
13. Senft C, Forster M-T, Bink A, Mittelbronn M, Franz K, Seifert V, et al. Optimizing the extent of resection in eloquently located gliomas by combining intraoperative MRI guidance with intraoperative neurophysiological monitoring. J Neurooncol. 2012;109:81-90.

14. Spetzler RF, Martin NA. A proposed grading system for arteriovenous malformations. J Neurosurg. 1986;65:476-83.
15. Jeong J-W, Asano E, Juhász C, Chugani HT. Localization of specific language pathways using diffusion-weighted imaging tractography for presurgical planning of children with intractable epilepsy. Epilepsia. 2015;56:49-57.
16. Jobst BC. Electrical stimulation in epilepsy: vagus nerve and brain stimulation. Curr Treat Options Neurol. 2010;12:443-53.
17. Asanuma H. Recent developments in the study of the columnar arrangement of neurons within the motor cortex. Physiol Rev. 1975;55:143-56.
18. Knecht S, Deppe M, Dräger B, Bobe L, Lohmann H, Ringelstein E, et al. Language lateralization in healthy right-handers. Brain J Neurol. 2000;123(Pt 1):74-81.
19. Korostenskaja M, Chen P-C, Salinas CM, Westerveld M, Brunner P, Schalk G, et al. Real-time functional mapping: potential tool for improving language outcome in pediatric epilepsy surgery. J Neurosurg Pediatr. 2014;14:287-95.
20. Lesser RP, Lüders H, Klem G, Dinner DS, Morris HH, Hahn JF, et al. Extraoperative cortical functional localization in patients with epilepsy. J Clin Neurophysiol. 1987;4:27-53.
21. Macewen W. An address on the surgery of the brain and spinal cord. Br Med J. 1888;2:302-9.
22. Magiorkinis E, Diamantis A, Sidiropoulou K, Panteliadis C. Highights in the history of epilepsy: the last 200 years. Epilepsy Res Treat. 2014;2014:1-13.
23. Meador KJ, Loring DW, Flanigin HF. History of epilepsy surgery. J Epilepsy. 1989;2:21-5.
24. Moo LR, Slotnick SD, Krauss G, Hart J. A prospective study of motor recovery following multiple subpial transections. Neuroreport. 2002;13:665-9.
25. Morrell F, Kanner A, Whisler W. Multiple subpial transection. In: Stefan H, Andermann F (Eds). Plasticity in Epilepsy. New York: Lippincott-Raven; 1998.
26. Morrell F, Whisler WW, Bleck TP. Multiple subpial transection: a new approach to the surgical treatment of focal epilepsy. J Neurosurg. 1989;70:231-9.
27. Mountcastle VB. Modality and topographic properties of single neurons of cat's somatic sensory cortex. J Neurophysiol. 1957;20:408-34.
28. Mountcastle VB. The columnar organization of the neocortex. Brain J Neurol. 1997;120(Pt 4):701-22.
29. Ojemann GA, Whitaker HA. Language localization and variability. Brain Lang. 1978;6:239-60.
30. Ojemann G, Ojemann J, Lettich E, Berger M. Cortical language localization in left, dominant hemisphere. An electrical stimulation mapping investigation in 117 patients. J Neurosurg. 1989;108:411-21.
31. Hagner M. The electrical excitability of the brain: toward the emergence of an experiment. J Hist Neurosci. 2012;21:237-49.
32. Orbach D, Romanelli P, Devinsky O, Doyle W. Late seizure recurrence after multiple subpial transections. Epilepsia. 2001;42:1316-9.
33. Reynolds E. Todd, Hughlings Jackson, and the electrical basis of epilepsy. Lancet. 2001;358:575-77.
34. Reynolds EH. Hughlings Jackson: a Yorkshireman's contribution to epilepsy. Arch Neurol. 1988;45:675.
35. Rezaie R, Narayana S, Schiller K, Birg L, Wheless JW, Boop FA, et al. Assessment of hemispheric dominance for receptive language in pediatric patients under sedation using magnetoencephalography. Front Hum Neurosci. 2014;8:657.
36. Schramm J, Aliashkevich AF, Grunwald T. Multiple subpial transections: outcome and complications in 20 patients who did not undergo resection. J Neurosurg. 2002;97:39-47.
37. Spencer SS, Schramm J, Wyler A, O'Connor M, Orbach D, Krauss G, et al. Multiple subpial transection for intractable partial epilepsy: an international meta-analysis. Epilepsia. 2002;43:141-5.
38. Hallett M. Transcranial magnetic stimulation and the human brain. Nature. 2000;406:147-50.
39. Springer JA, Binder JR, Hammeke TA, Swanson SJ, Frost JA, Bellgowan PS, et al. Language dominance in neurologically normal and epilepsy subjects: a functional MRI study. Brain J Neurol. 1999;122(Pt 11):2033-46.

40. Suarez RO, Taimouri V, Boyer K, Vega C, Rotenberg A, Madsen JR, et al: Passive fMRI mapping of language function for pediatric epilepsy surgical planning: validation using Wada, ECS, and FMAER. Epilepsy Res. 2014;108:1874-88.
41. Sun FT, Morrell MJ. Closed-loop neurostimulation: the clinical experience. Neurotherapeutics. 2014;11:553-63.
42. Whisler W. Multiple subpial transection. In: Neurosurgical Operative Atlas. Park Ridge, IL: American Association of Neurological Surgeons; 1997. pp. 125-9.
43. Whisler W. Multiple subpial transection. In: Kaye A, Black P (Eds). Operative Neurosurgery. United Kingdom: Churchill Livingstone; 1997.
44. Child ND, Stead M, Wirrell EC, Nickels KC, Wetjen NM, Lee KH, et al. Chronic subthreshold subdural cortical stimulation for the treatment of focal epilepsy originating from eloquent cortex. Epilepsia. 2014;55:e18-21.
45. DiLorenzo DJ, Mangubat EZ, Rossi MA, Byrne RW. Chronic unlimited recording electrocorticography-guided resective epilepsy surgery: technology-enabled enhanced fidelity in seizure focus localization with improved surgical efficacy. J Neurosurg. 2014;120:1402-14.

CHAPTER

9

Surgery for Giant and Unusual Tumors of the Limbic System

Sahin Hanalioglu, Ilhan Aydin, Ulas Cikla, Mustafa K Baskaya

INTRODUCTION

The limbic system consists of complex structures located between diencephalon and telencephalon. Occupying medial and basal parts of hemispheres, it comprises of both cortical and subcortical elements. Cortical regions involved in the limbic system including the hippocampus, parahippocampal gyrus, cingulate gyrus (CG), subcallosal gyrus and orbital frontal cortex—altogether form the so-called "limbic lobe", the term coined by Broca in 1878 (Fig. 9.1).[1] This cortex surrounds the corpus callosum like a rim. Subcortical and diencephalic elements of the limbic system include the olfactory bulb, hypothalamus, amygdala, septal

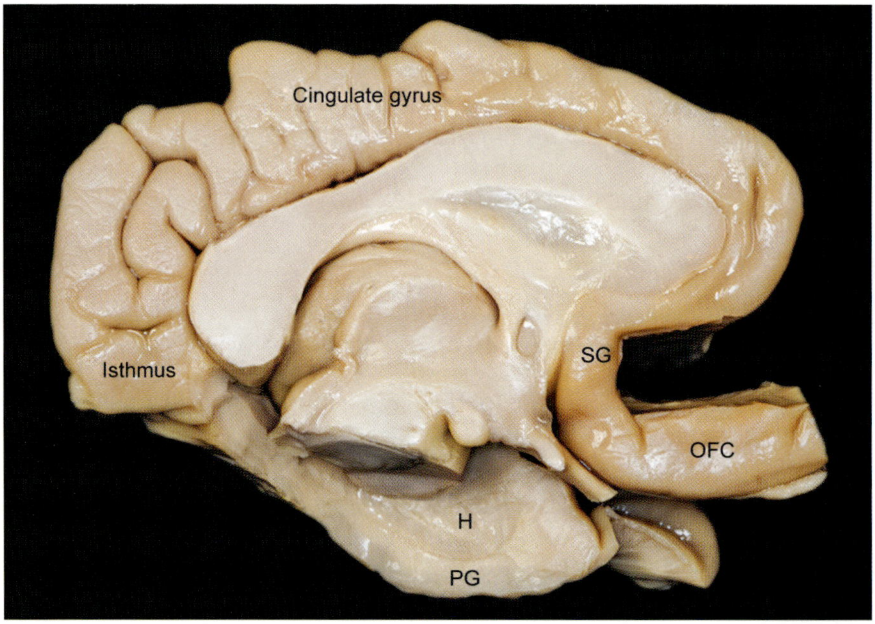

Fig. 9.1: Cadaveric dissection shows structures of the limbic lobe including the hippocampus, parahippocampal, cingulate, subcallosal gyri, and orbital frontal cortex.
(SG: Subcallosal gyrus; OFC: Orbitofrontal cortex; H: Hippocampus; PG: Parahippocampal gyrus).

nuclei, mammillary bodies, nucleus accumbens and anterior thalamic nuclei. Recently, limbic lobe has been redefined to incorporate the extended amygdala and ventral striatopallidal system among the limbic output channels.[2]

In 1937, Papez proposed a neural circuit, connecting the hypothalamus to the limbic lobe, for the control of emotional expression.[3] Later in 1952, MacLean modified the circuit and coined the term "limbic system" for limbic cortex and associated brainstem structures.[4] The limbic system is considered as an interface between subcortical structures and cerebral cortex. With its complex functional and anatomical connections within the entire nervous system, it is highly involved in learning, memory, motivation, emotion, behavior and autonomic/visceral responses.[5]

From an evolutionary and embryological standpoint, limbic system has a distinct place among other brain structures. During the evolutionary march of the mammalian brain, the limbic lobe is thought to emerge after so-called "reptilian brain" composed of the brainstem and striatal nuclei and before highly convoluted, phylogenetically younger neocortex.[4,6] Limbic structures or allocortex are the most primitive cortex and include septal regions, substantia innominata, and amygdala (no lamination) or hippocampal and piriform cortex (two layer lamination). Paralimbic structures or mesocortex includes caudal orbitofrontal cortex, insula, temporal pole, parahippocampal and cingulate gyri and have three to five cortical layers. Indeed, mesocortical structures connect allocortical structures to the six-layered neocortex and are anatomically placed between those two domains. Vascularization of limbic and paralimbic areas also parallels anatomic and histological development; their arterial supply and venous drainage are via both superficial and deep vascular systems as opposed to central (reptilian) and neocortical areas.[6]

Once considered inoperable lesions, limbic and paralimbic tumors drew attention among neurosurgeons only after the early 1990s, when the first extensive series of microsurgically treated limbic and paralimbic tumors were reported by Yasargil.[6,7] In his seminal paper, Yasargil described clinical and radiological features and surgical outcomes of 177 patients with tumors of the mediobasal temporal, insular, temporal pole-anterior insular-orbitofrontal areas out of a total of 240 patients with limbic and paralimbic tumors.[6] Yasargil classified intrinsic tumors within the limbic and paralimbic regions based on location, and he later modified this classification slightly (Tables 9.1 and 9.2).[7] He divided limbic and paralimbic areas into four primary regions: (1) mediobasal temporal, (2) cingulate gyrus, (3) insula, and (4) orbitofrontal lobe (Tables 9.1 and 9.2).

Yasargil noted that surgical and clinical features of mediobasal temporal, insular, orbitofrontal-insular-temporal pole tumors have striking similarities from clinical and surgical viewpoints, and they represent a distinct variety of brain tumors.[6] Following this study, the microsurgical anatomy of limbic/paralimbic areas has been investigated in detail by various authors from the perspectives of epilepsy, tumor or arteriovenous malformation (AVM) surgery.[8-15] Also, some large clinical series of tumors involving limbic and paralimbic structures have been reported in the literature.[7,16-20] Here, we summarize relevant microsurgical anatomy, clinical and pathological features, surgical approaches to and outcomes of the tumors arising from the mediobasal temporal region and CG with a particular emphasis on large/giant tumors. We also present some illustrative cases and selected surgical techniques to approach those tumors.

Table 9.1: Yasargil's anatomical classification of limbic and paralimbic regions.[7]	
1. Mediobasal temporal (1a–c) and associated limbic structures (1d–g)	
a.	Temporal pole (medial)
b.	Amygdala with the stria terminalis
c.	Uncus/hippocampus/parahippocampus
d.	Indusium griseum
e.	Fornix
f.	Mammillary body
g.	Septal nuclei
2. Cingulate gyrus	
a.	Anterior
b.	Middle
c.	Posterior
3. Insula	
4. Fronto-orbital and subcallosal areas	

Table 9.2: Yasargil's classification of limbic and paralimbic tumors based on location.[7]	
1. Temporal mediobasal	
a.	Temporal pole (medial)
b.	Amygdala
c.	Hippocampus
d.	Parahippocampus
2. Cingulate gyrus	
a.	Anterior
b.	Middle
c.	Posterior
3. Insula and parainsula	
a.	Pure insula
b.	Insular-frontobasal
c.	Insular-temporal mediobasal
d.	Insular-frontobasal-septal and temporal mediobasal
4. Medial limbic association areas	
a.	Fornix
b.	Septal areas
c.	Mammillary body
5. Entire limbic system (areas 1–4)	

MEDIOBASAL TEMPORAL TUMORS

An Overview of Microsurgical Anatomy

Mediobasal temporal (MBT) region comprises of essential elements of the limbic system and is closely related to vital structures medially such as cerebral peduncles and the circle of Willis. It contains both intraventricular and extraventricular elements which are closely related. The intraventricular elements are the hippocampus, amygdala, fimbria, and choroidal fissure; while the extraventricular elements include the parahippocampal gyrus, uncus and dentate gyrus. Temporal stem constitutes an elaborate white and gray matter bridge between the temporal lobe and deep structures such as insula, basal ganglia, and diencephalon. The parahippocampal gyrus extends from uncus anteriorly to the isthmus of the CG posteriorly and continues as the lingual gyrus. The parahippocampal gyrus is limited by the collateral (posterior) and rhinal (anterior) sulci laterally (Fig. 9.2), and the parahippocampal gyrus is related to the edge of the tentorium and the neurovascular content of the ambient cistern medially.

The hippocampus forms a comma like an arc, occupies the medial floor of the temporal horn and consists of three parts: (1) head, (2) body, and (3) tail (Fig. 9.3). Superiorly, the head of the hippocampus is related to the posteroinferior portion of the amygdala. The head of the hippocampus constitutes the anterior third of the medial wall, while the choroidal fissure forms the posterior two-thirds of the medial wall of temporal horn. Posteriorly, the body

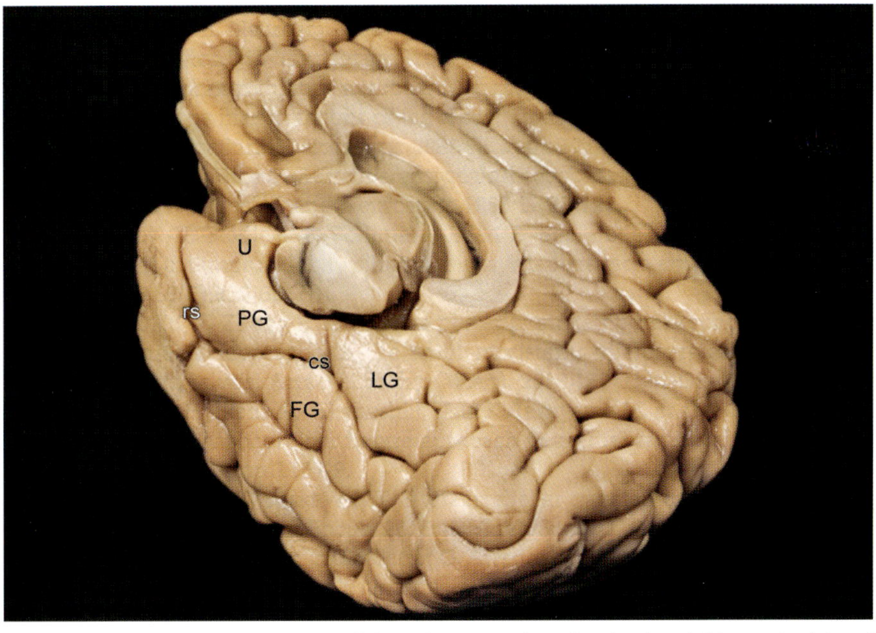

Fig. 9.2: The inferomedial view of the mediobasal temporal region in the right cerebral hemisphere is shown in a cadaveric brain.
(U: Uncus; PG: Parahippocampal gyrus; LG: Lingual gyrus; FG: Fusiform gyrus; rs: Rhinal sulcus; cs: Collateral sulcus).

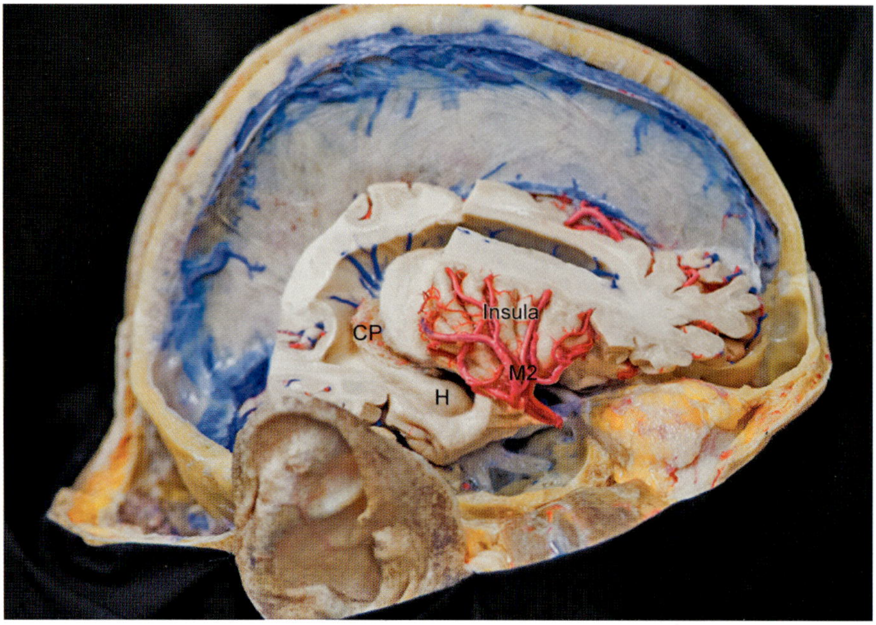

Fig. 9.3: Lateral view of the hippocampus and insula with relationship of the middle cerebral artery. (H: Hippocampus; CP: Choroid plexus; M2: Insular segment of the middle cerebral artery).

of the hippocampus narrows as it approaches the atrium of the lateral ventricle. The tail of the hippocampus constitutes the medial part of the floor of the atrium and continues as the subsplenial gyrus. Posterior and superior to the uncus is the inferior choroidal point, where the choroid plexus of the temporal horn begins, anterior choroidal artery (AChoA) enters and the inferior ventricular vein leaves the temporal horn through the choroidal fissure.

Arterial supply of MBT structures is mainly from AChoA and posterior cerebral artery (PCA). Lateral posterior choroidal artery (PChoA) from P2 segment and AChoA anastomose within the temporal horn. The inferior temporal arteries arising from PCA include the hippocampal artery, anterior, middle, and posterior temporal arteries. The anterior temporal artery arises mainly from P2A, whereas the middle and posterior temporal arteries arise mostly from the P2P segment. Early branches of M1 also supply temporal pole. The deep venous system of the MBT region drains into the basal vein of Rosenthal.

Clinical Features of MBT Tumors

Mediobasal temporal tumors appear to occur in relatively younger age. In Yasargil's series, 60% of the patients were under 40 years old. In Schramm's large series of 235 MBT tumor patients, the mean age at diagnosis was 35 years. Other authors also reported similar average age at presentation (30–50 years).[7,16,20] A male preponderance (M-to-F ratio: 1.3–1.6) was observed by various authors.[7,16,20] In most of the published series, the prominent symptom of MBT tumors are seizures (52–94%),[6,20] except for one series reporting intracranial hypertension as the primary clinical manifestation (66%). Drug-resistant epilepsy lasting longer than 2 years was present in 78% of the patients in of the largest published series.[17] Partial seizures comprise the majority of the seizures encountered in MBT tumor patients.[6,17] Preoperative neurological deficits are not so common and appear to be mild in most cases. In Yasargil's series, more than half of the patients had no mental or neurological deficits.

Growth Patterns and Anatomical Classifications

Limbic and paralimbic tumors may exhibit various growth patterns as detected by high-resolution magnetic resonance imaging (MRI). Those tumors may stay limited in a subregion, grow within a region or spread to adjacent areas. Interestingly most limbic tumors tend to spread within the boundaries of allocortical or mesocortical regions but not invading neighboring neocortex and medial structures such as basal ganglia and internal capsule until tumor acquires a more malignant and aggressive behavior in the advanced stage.[6] Gliomas in the limbic and paralimbic systems, preferentially extend along white matter tracts.[21] A radiological study investigating low-grade gliomas centered on the insula and extending into temporal and frontal lobes found that 70% of the tumors (mainly frontal-orbital-insular-temporal pole) spread along uncinate fasciculus while a lower percentage of the tumors of this region preferred arcuate fasciculus, inferior fronto-occipital fasciculus, and optic radiations (Fig. 9.4).[21-24] Another study showed gliomas confined within any of the paralimbic regions (fronto-orbital, insular, temporal pole) would eventually grow to involve all three parts during a dynamic radiological examination over time.[25-28] MBT tumors may also spread through fornix and cingulate fasciculus. In Yasargil's series, the growth of parahippocampal tumors toward posterior CG was observed in some cases. Entire limbic/paralimbic system involvement could also be seen rarely.

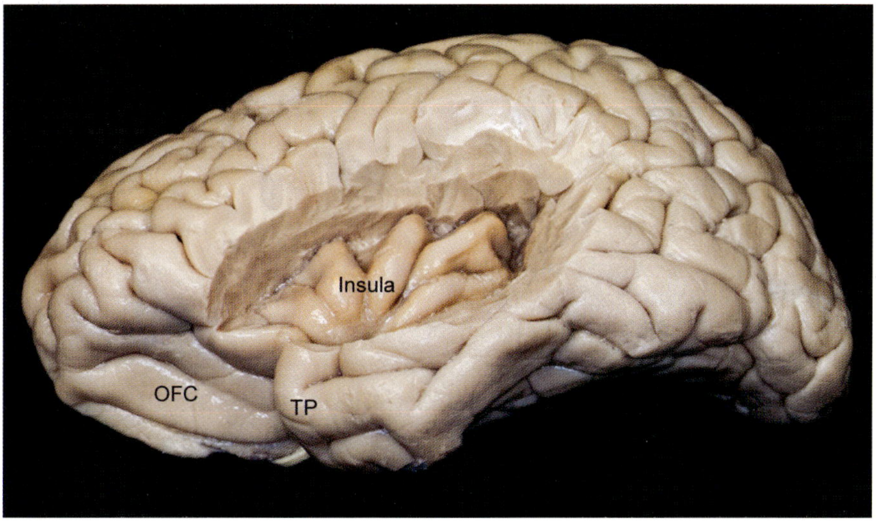

Fig. 9.4: Superior and middle temporal gyri have been removed to expose the insular cortex. Inferolateral view of the paralimbic regions (fronto-orbital, insula and temporal pole).
(OFC: Orbitofrontal cortex; TP: Temporal pole).

While Yasargil's classification was based on the compartmentalization of the full range of limbic/paralimbic tumors, classification proposed by Schramm and Aliashkevich[16] took consideration anatomical landmarks. According to their classification, type A tumors arise from the mediobasal structures (amygdala, hippocampus, parahippocampus and lingual gyrus). Type B tumors are located lateral to the collateral sulcus without extension into the inferior and medial temporal gyri. Type C tumors are the combination of type A and B. Type D tumors can start as A, B or C with extension into the basal ganglia or subcortical insular area through the temporal stem. As implied, types C and D tumors comprise the majority of large/giant MBT tumors (83% of the tumors >5 cm) as compared with types A and B among which large/giant tumors account for less than 5%. An important difference between Schramm's and Yasargil's series is that almost two-thirds of tumors in Yasargil's series were larger than 5 cm in size whereas only 12% of Schramm's series were large tumors.[29]

Histopathological Characteristics

Neuroepithelial tumors account for vast majority of MBT tumors. In contrary to other brain regions, metastases of the limbic circuit are uncommon. Only 5% of all metastases were encountered in the limbic system.[30] In accordance, only 1% of MBT tumors were metastases in Schramm's series. In Yasargil's series, half of the all limbic and paralimbic tumors and 57% of MBT tumors were benign. Three most common MBT tumors were grade I–II ganglioglioma (21%), grade I–II astrocytoma (18%) and grade III astrocytoma (17%). In another large series, 47% had grade I, 29% grade II, 10% grade III and 11% grade IV tumors. Similarly, grade I ganglioglioma (28%), grade II astrocytoma (13%) and grade IV glioblastoma (11%) were the most common histopathological diagnoses. However, malignant tumors comprised only 24% of this series.[17] As reflected in the frequency of gangliogliomas, neuronal differentiation is more frequent in MBT tumors than other limbic and extralimbic tumors, possibly due to the proximity to the subgranular zone of the dentate gyrus.

There are only a few studies exploring molecular fingerprints of the MBT tumors. One study was comparing mediobasal and lateral temporal gliomas (LTG), found no differences in 1p/19q codeletion, polysomy, MGMT promoter methylation or the expression of 12 tumor-associated proteins between two groups. However, slightly higher rate of IDH1/2 mutations was detected in LTG group.[20] It is well-established that pure insular gliomas almost exclusively harbor IDH1/2 mutations. However, paralimbic gliomas exhibit a lower rate of IDH1/2 mutations.[31,32]

Surgery of MBT Tumors

Surgical Approaches

Yasargil advocated for pterional craniotomy with transsylvian approach without the need for a cortical incision or temporal lobectomy for the entire range of MBT, insular or parainsular tumors except for a few posteriorly extended ones. In his technique, the opening of anterior two-thirds of Sylvian fissure exposes the internal carotid artery (ICA) and M1 bifurcations, 1–2 cm of M2 segments, superficial and deep Sylvian veins and their tributaries. After the identification of inferior limiting insular sulcus at the level of limen insula, a 1–2 cm incision is

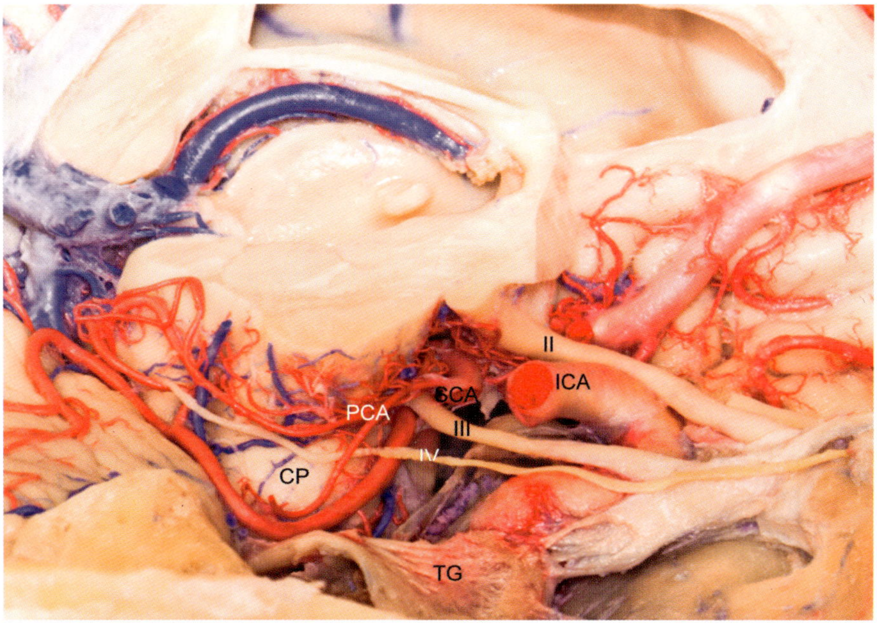

Fig. 9.5: Cadaveric dissection demonstrates neurovascular structures after limbic and paralimbic structures have been removed.
(PCA: Posterior cerebral artery; SCA: Superior cerebellar artery; ICA: Internal cerebral artery; CP: Cerebral peduncle; TG: Trigeminal ganglion; II: Optic nerve; III: Oculomotor nerve; IV: Trochlear nerve).

made lateral to the inferior circumferential insular vein, and the temporal horn is opened at a depth of 1–1.5 cm. In his experience, larger tumors are easier to extirpate due to so-called "birth channel" developed around slowly growing a tumor. For the large tumors, a central decompression by first removing anterosuperiorly, then central portions of the tumor, is required to be able to open the choroidal fissure and recognize the vital neurovascular structures such as optic tract, cranial nerves III–IV, cerebral peduncle, P1-P2-P3 branches, posterior communicating artery (PCoA), AChoA, PChoA and basal vein (Fig. 9.5). Small arterial feeders mainly from AChoA, P2, and P3 can be coagulated to reduce blood supply of the tumor. Therefore, total tumor resection can be achieved anteroposteriorly even as far as trigone and posterior pole of incisura. However, if the tumor is extended more posteriorly (e.g. into posterior CG), the second operation via posterior interhemispheric approach is needed.

Despite Yasargil's successful surgical technique and favorable results, various authors have since attempted to use both classical and newly described methods to be able to maximize the extent of resection while preserving function to the fullest extent. Schramm utilized his anatomical classification to describe the preferred use of individual approaches for different tumor types. Hence, the most frequently adopted approaches were transsylvian for type A; subtemporal for type B; anterior two-thirds temporal lobe resection for type C and type D tumors. Anterior temporal lobectomy (or anterior two-thirds resection) was preferred in 38%, followed by subtemporal in 24% and transsylvian in 16% for type C and D tumors [including 83% of large (>5 cm) tumors], collectively. In general, anteriorly located tumors can be accessed and entirely

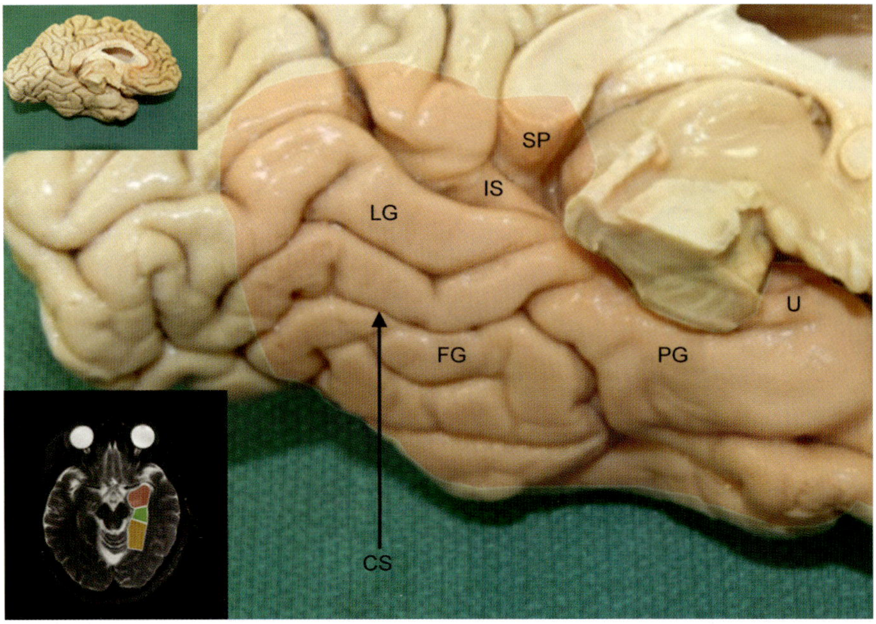

Fig. 9.6: Cadaveric dissection of the left hemisphere and T2 axial MRI show an imaginary division of the mediobasal temporal region into three regions. The anterior one-third begins from the uncus and ends of the junction of crural and ambient cisterns. The middle-third ends at the junction of ambient and quadrigeminal cisterns. The posterior one-third includes quadrigeminal cistern and lingual gyrus.
(LG: Lingual gyrus; FG: Fusiform gyrus; PG: Parahippocampal gyrus; U: Uncus; SP: Splenium; IS: Isthmus; CS: Collateral sulcus).

removed via a transsylvian or standard anterior cortical resection with or without hippocampectomy depending on epileptological reasons or tumor type. However, posterior MBT tumors pose challenges, if approached via transsylvian route particularly in the setting of small tumors. Therefore, Schramm advocates for subtemporal approach with or without small basal gyrus resection and its modifications for those types of tumors. He also notes that large tumors in the posterior dominant temporal lobe have potential risks of causing language problems, if approached via a subtemporal route.[33]

In addition to surgical approaches proposed by Yasargil and Schramm, several other authors have described alternative surgical approaches to reach various parts of the MBT region. These include various transcortical approaches,[34-37] low posterior transtemporal approaches after petrosectomy,[38,39] occipital interhemispheric approach[21,40] and supracerebellar transtentorial approach.[41,42] Posterior approaches including supratentorial infraoccipital/posterior interhemispheric[7,40] and paramedian supracerebellar-transtentorial[38,41-44] approaches. Each approach has its advantages and disadvantages in reaching to various parts of the MBT region.[45]

In selecting surgical approach, we prefer to divide entire mediobasal region into three imaginary regions (Fig. 9.6). If the tumor is small and only involves one of these three regions, we use transsylvian approach for lesions located in the anterior one-third segment of the MBT

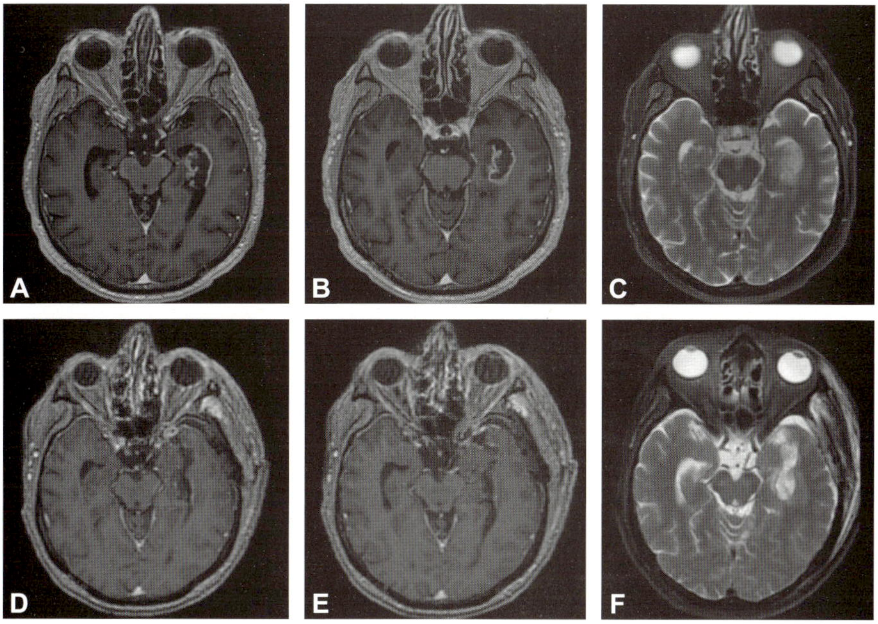

Figs. 9.7A to F: MRI of a 78-year-old male patient who presented with complex partial seizures. Preoperative T1-postcontrast axial (A and B) and T2 axial (C) MRIs show heterogeneously enhancing tumor in the anterior one-third of the mediobasal region within the temporal horn of the lateral ventricle. Postoperative T1 postcontrast axial (D and E) and T2 axial (F) MRIs show gross total resection of grade IV astrocytoma via transsylvian transuncal approach.

region (Figs. 9.7A to F), subtemporal approach for lesions in the middle-third (Figs. 9.8A to F) and supracerebellar transtentorial approach for lesions in the posterior-third (*see* Chapter 4 "Supracerebellar Transtentorial Approach to Limbic Tumors"). The lesions spanning anterior and middle regions can be reached via transsylvian approach while those involving both middle and posterior regions can be accessed with supracerebellar transtentorial approach. For tumors involving anterior one-third with extension into the temporal pole, temporal polectomy with transsylvian approach would be preferred (Figs. 9.9A and B). For those tumors that involve entire mediobasal region with or without extension into the posterior CG through isthmus, multiple stage surgeries utilizing more than one approach might be necessary (Figs. 9.10A to D).

We also favor of using multiple stage surgeries regardless of the involvement of various areas in some large or giant limbic tumors to avoid problems many arise from long hours of surgery (Figs. 9.11A to F).

Surgical Outcomes

In general, microsurgery yields favorable results regarding overall and progression-free survival, preservation of function and epilepsy control.[46] Yasargil reported that surgery led to good postoperative conditions in 95% and fair in 5% of benign tumors, while 76.5% of

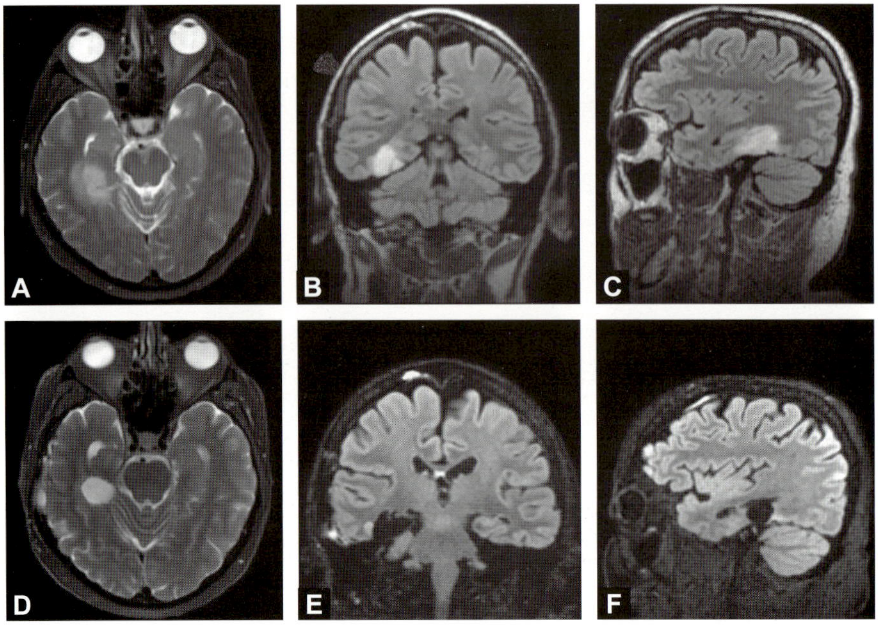

Figs. 9.8A to F: MRI of a 58-year-old male who presented with seizures. Preoperative T2 axial (A), T2 flair-cube coronal (B) and sagittal (C) MRIs show tumor involving the medial one-third of the mediobasal temporal region. Postoperative T2 axial (D), T2 flair-cube coronal (E) and sagittal (F) MRIs show gross total resection of grade III astrocytoma via subtemporal approach.

malignant tumors had good conditions. He had no operative mortality or serious morbidity. However, all malignant but only 7.5% of benign tumors recurred during follow-up. Excellent seizure control was achieved in 77% (Engel class I: No seizures) of benign tumor group.[7] Schramm also reported good operative results. However, he also underlines surgical complications associated with different approaches. In his large series, the most common temporary complications include speech disturbances (6.0%), hemiparesis (5.1%) and meningitis (5.1%). Permanent complications include significant visual field defects (hemianopia) (5.4%) and severe sequelae (1.7%) along with one operative mortality (0.4%). Other published series also have similar figures. Postoperative worsening of visual field defects was seen in the form of quadrantanopia in 14–36% and hemianopia 3–10%.[7,17,36,47] Away all published series, there was no significant difference in the primary complications between transsylvian and classic anterior two-thirds lobe resection.

CINGULATE GYRUS TUMORS

An Overview of Anatomy

The cingulate gyrus is C-shaped cortical structure lying on the medial surface of the cerebral hemispheres. It begins from the lamina terminalis (subcallosal cortex), extends above corpus callosum posteriorly, goes around the splenium, and finally joins with parahippocampal gyrus

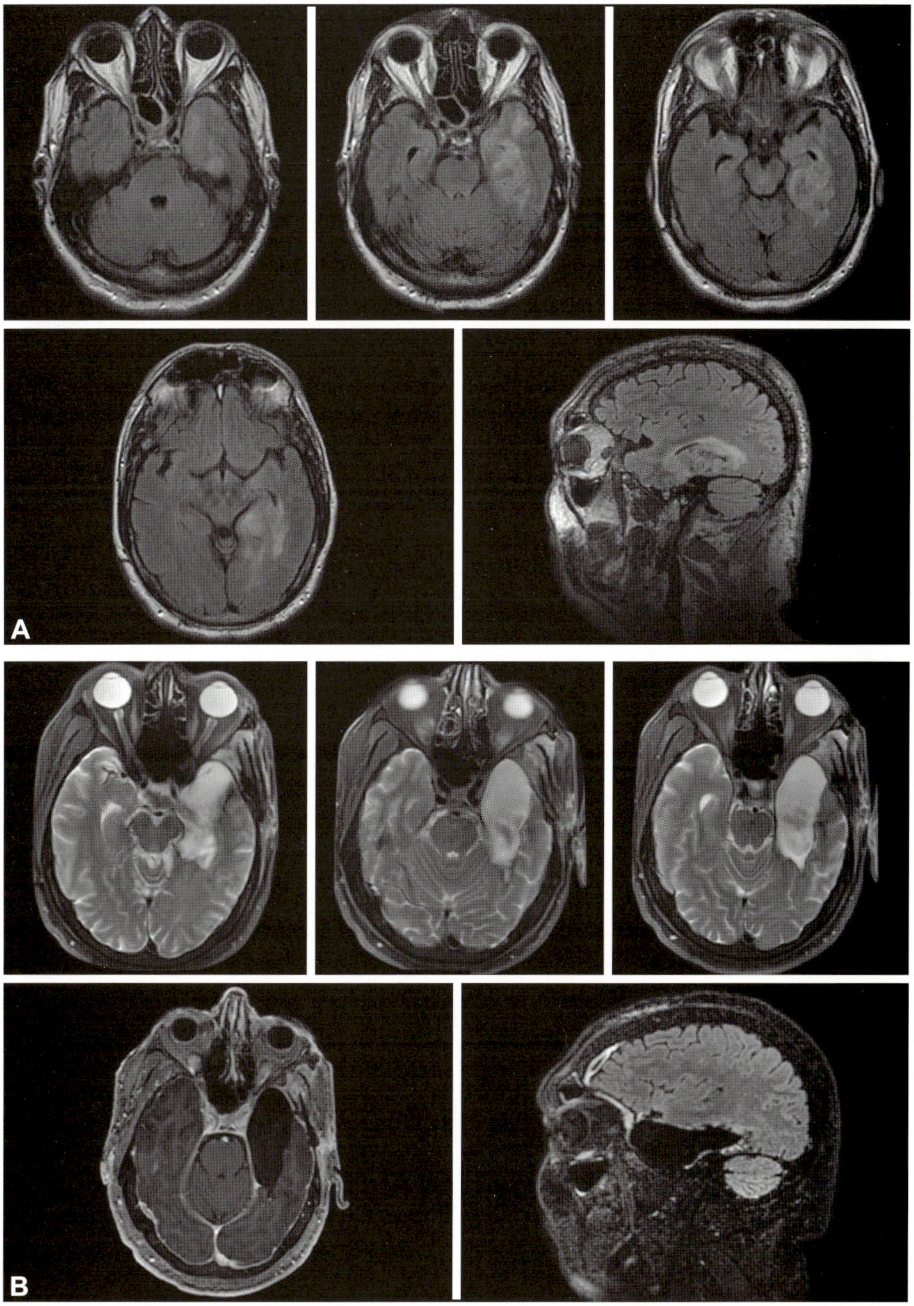

Figs. 9.9A and B: MRI of a 62-year-old male who presented with complex partial seizures. Preoperative T2 flair-cube axial and sagittal MRIs show large to giant size (7 cm in size) tumor involving the anterior and middle thirds of the mediobasal region with extension into the temporal pole (A). Postoperative T2 and T1-postcontrast axial and sagittal flair-cube (B) MRIs show gross total resection of grade II astrocytoma via transsylvian approach with temporal polectomy. The patient made an excellent recovery without any speech or memory problems.

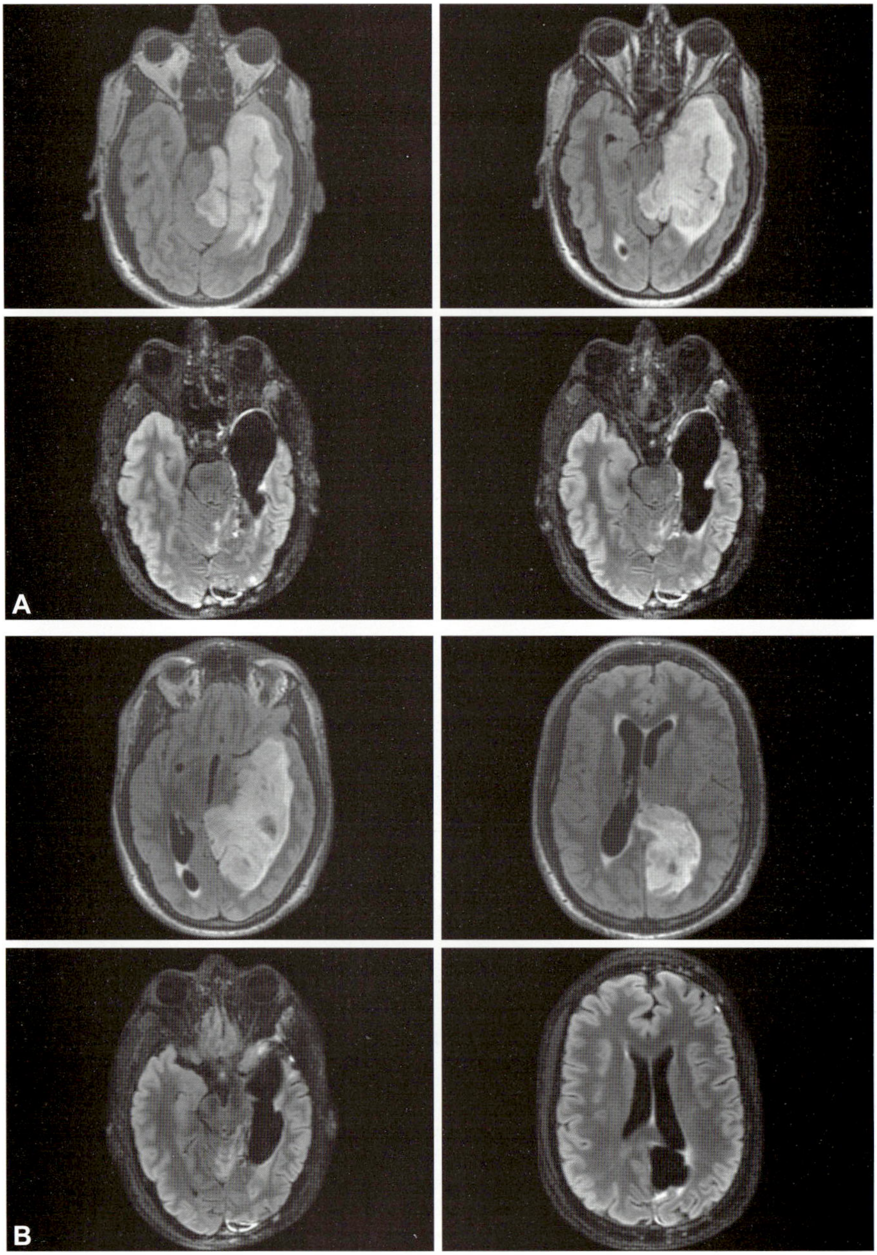

Figs. 9.10A and B

through the isthmus. It is considered an integral part of the limbic system and has complex anatomical and functional connections with various brain structures such as the thalamus, hippocampus, amygdala, insula, orbitofrontal and premotor cortices. The CG is surrounded superiorly by superior frontal gyrus, paracentral lobule and precuneus from anterior to posterior.

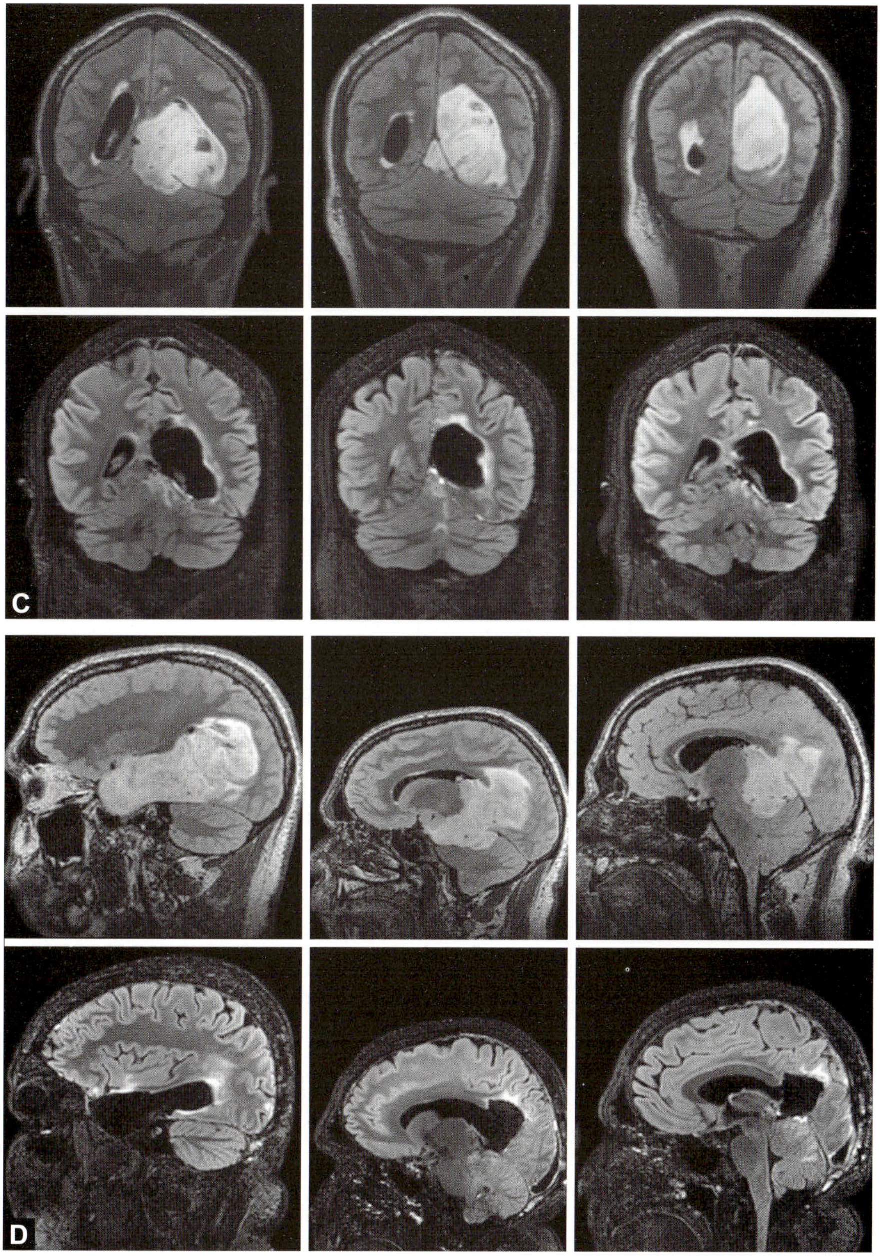

Figs. 9.10A to D: MRI of a 36-year-old male who presented with confusion, speech problems and lack of concentration. Preoperative T2 flair-cube axial (upper panel of A and B), coronal (upper panel of C) and sagittal (upper panel of D) MRIs show giant tumor involving entire mediobasal temporal region (from the temporal pole and uncus to posterior parahippocampal gyrus to posterior cingulate gyrus). The patient underwent three-stage surgery in an order as follows. (1) transsylvian approaches with temporal polectomy, (2) supracerebellar transtentorial approach and (3) occipital interhemispheric approach. He made an excellent recovery with return to his premorbid baseline. Pathology was grade II astrocytoma.

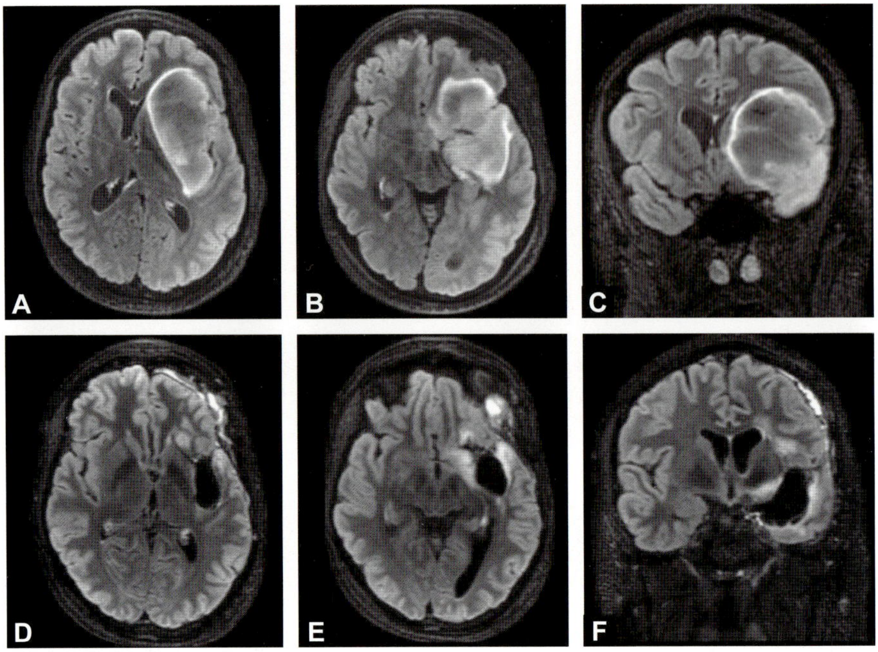

Figs. 9.11A to F: MRI scan of a 24-year-old male who presented with complex partial seizures. Preoperative flair-cube axial (A and B) and coronal (C) MRIs show giant, approximately 7 cm tumor in the left insula. The patient underwent transsylvian resection of the tumor with motor evoked potential monitoring. Due to long hours of surgery at the first stage, a decision was made to come back in 2 days for the definitive second stage. Postoperative flair-cube axial (D and E) and coronal (F) MRIs show gross total or near-total resection of grade II astrocytoma. The patient made an excellent recovery without any permanent speech problems.

Pericallosal arteries arise from ACA and travel over the corpus callosum to anastomose with posterior pericallosal arteries originating from PCA (Fig. 9.12).

Clinical Features of Cingulate Gyrus Tumors

There have been a few published series of CG tumors. It is thought that CG gliomas constitute 3–5% of all supratentorial gliomas. Mean age at the diagnosis is reported to be 39–48 years.[7,18,19,48,49] Some studies found a slight male predominance[18,48,49] whereas the others did not.[7,19] The most common initial symptom is seizures (55–85%) followed by motor and speech deficits, headache and psychiatric disturbances. Preoperative hemiparesis can be seen in 7–17% of the patients. Although strongly implicated in mental disorders such as schizophrenia and anxiety, interestingly severe psychiatric symptoms are not so common in CG tumors.

Anatomical Classification and Growth Patterns

Classically, CG is divided into two major parts, (1) anterior and (2) posterior, according to the central sulcus. Yasargil used a different system which divided CG into three sections: (1) anterior, (2) middle and (3) posterior.

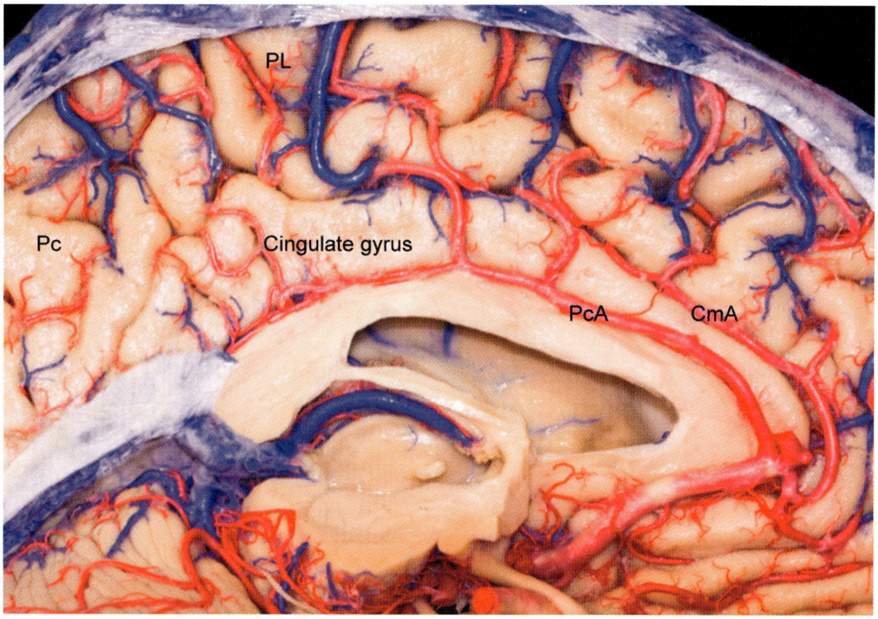

Fig. 9.12: Cadaveric dissection demonstrates entire cingulate gyrus with surrounding gyri and vascular structures.
(Pc: Precuneus; PL: Paracentral lobule; PcA: Pericallosal artery; CmA: Callosomarginal artery).

Cingulate gyrus tumors may be confined to the CG or expand to adjacent structures. Tumors solely located in the CG represent roughly 30–40% of all CG tumors.[18,19,48] In the remaining cases, tumor (mainly glioma) may infiltrate supracingular structures, fronto-orbital cortex, insula, or mediobasal temporal region. Growth patterns usually follow anatomical connections of CG: anterior cingulate tumors extend into septal and dorsomedial superior frontal gyrus; middle cingulate tumors to paracentral and precuneal gyri, and posterior cingulate tumors to parahippocampal gyrus and precuneus.[7] Infiltration of the corpus callosum is also frequent (42%).[48] Expansion towards lateral ventricles and septum pellucidum are also observed in large tumors. Von Leve et al. (2009) and Oszvald et al. (2012) used classical (two-region) classification and reported that 82% and 86% of CG tumors occurred in anterior CG. In Yasargil's series, however, anterior CG accounted for 30%, middle CG for 24%, posterior CG for 46% of all cingulate tumors. Unfortunately, most of the published CG tumor series do not provide information about tumor size. Yasargil reported that 63% in his series of 54 CG tumors were larger than 5 cm in diameter. In the two separate series of anterior and posterior CG tumors by the same group, the tumors larger than 4 cm comprised 84% and 49% of the respective series.[50,51]

Histopathological Characteristics

Tumors involving CG are almost exclusively glial origin. The majority of the tumors are malignant (grade III–IV) with varying rates in the published series (50–75%). Grade I–II tumors represented 25–49% of all tumors whereas grade IIIs were 26–64%, grade IVs were 18–49%.[7,18,19,48,49]

Most commonly seen pathologies were glioblastoma (17–49%), anaplastic mixed oligoastrocytoma (6–36%), mixed oligoastrocytoma (5–27%), anaplastic astrocytoma (8–21%), diffuse astrocytoma (9–17%), oligodendroglioma (3–18%).[7,18,19,48,49] Interestingly, in contrast to the mediobasal temporal limbic tumors, the oligodendroglial component becomes more frequent (27–46%) while the neuronal component is less commonly seen in the tumors of this region (0–13%).

Surgery of Cingulate Gyrus Tumors

Surgical Approaches

The interhemispheric approach is the preferred surgical routes for the vast majority of the CG tumors, but, in particular, for pure cingulate gliomas.[7,48] In the event of a supracingular extension, however, a transcortical approach might be more feasible if tumor reaches the cortical surface. For an interhemispheric approach, an appropriate craniotomy large enough in anterior-posterior orientation is recommended to avoid damage to bridging veins or overretraction of motor cortex.[48] Since the tumor expansion over the corpus callosum and pericallosal arteries is quite common, central decompression in a subpial fashion is necessary to avoid injury to these arteries. Once the medial pial surface of the CG reached, pericallosal arteries can be identified, and then tumor feeders can be coagulated and cut to achieve total removal of the tumor.[7,10,52] Although Yasargil exclusively used interhemispheric approach for the entire range of cingulate tumors successfully; Berger and his colleagues, as well as Schramm, achieved comparable results with the transcortical approach with large and laterally-extended tumors with the aid of intraoperative electrophysiological mapping and neuronavigation.[18,48]

Talacchi used variations of interhemispheric approaches including unilateral interhemispheric, bilateral interhemispheric, unilateral interhemispheric + gyrectomy, unilateral interhemispheric + polectomy for anterior cingulate tumors depending on tumor location, extension pattern and pathology.[50] Alternative approaches to CG tumors include supracerebellar-transtentorial approach for posterior CG lesions and contralateral transcingulate approach for lesions near eloquent cortices.[10,53]

Surgical Outcomes

Although there is a discrepancy between the definitions of total resection for the CG tumors in the published literature, various authors reported gross total resection rates between 66% and 91%. Yasargil reported a good outcome for 92% of benign and 47% of malignant gliomas. He noted that the patients with poor surgical results in the malignant group were those already in worse clinical conditions preoperatively. Seventeen percent in the benign group and all in the malignant group recurred during follow-up in his series. Steiger et al. and Oszvald et al. observed a trend toward a more favorable prognosis than all other frontal gliomas. Furthermore, the patients with CG-only gliomas seem to have even higher survival rates than those with tumor extension beyond anatomical borders of CG.[19]

A few studies focused on surgical morbidity and functional outcome.[18,19,48] The most common postoperative morbidity is supplementary motor area (SMA) syndrome (14–34%) among all postoperative morbidity (15–40%). SMA syndrome is encountered in anterior CG tumors and thought to be related to surgical trajectory rather than cingulate resection itself.[18] Sensorimotor disturbances may occur after resection of the tumors in Zones II and III, which are in proximity to the motor and sensory cortices.[18] The majority of the early postoperative functional deficits improve with time, and long-term morbidity is only around 5% with various surgical approaches.[7,18,19.]

REFERENCES

1. Broca P. Anatomie comparee des circonvolutions cerebrales: Le grand lobe limbique et la scissure limbique dans la serie des mammiferes. Rev Anthrop. 1878;1:385-498.
2. Heimer L, Van Hoesen GW. The limbic lobe and its output channels: implications for emotional functions and adaptive behavior. Neurosci Biobehav Rev. 2006;30(2):126-47.
3. Papez JW. A proposed mechanism of emotion. Arch Neurol Psychiatry. 1937;38(4):725-43.
4. MacLean PD. The triune brain in evolution: Role in paleocerebral functions. Germany, Berlin: Springer Science & Business Media; 1990.
5. Nieuwenhuys R, Voogd J, Van Huijzen C. The Human Central Nervous System: A Synopsis and Atlas. Germany, Berlin: Springer Science & Business Media; 2007.
6. Yaşargil MG, Reeves JD. Tumours of the limbic and paralimbic system. Acta Neurochir (Wien). 1992;116(2-4):147-9.
7. Yaşargil MG. Limbic and paralimbic tumors. In: Yaşargil MG (Ed). Microneurosurgery, Vol. IVB. New York: Thieme; 1996. pp. 252-90.
8. Wen HT, Rhoton AL Jr, de Oliveira E, Cardoso AC, Tedeschi H, Baccanelli M, et al. Microsurgical anatomy of the temporal lobe: part 1: mesial temporal lobe anatomy and its vascular relationships as applied to amygdalohippocampectomy. Neurosurgery. 1999;45(3):549-91; discussion 591-2.
9. Türe U, Yaşargil DC, Al-Mefty O, Yaşargil MG. Topographic anatomy of the insular region. J Neurosurg. 1999;90(4):720-33.
10. Yaşargil MG, Türe U, Yaşargil DC. Surgical anatomy of supratentorial midline lesions. Neurosurg Focus. 2005;18(6B):E1.
11. Fernández-Miranda JC, de Oliveira E, Rubino PA, Wen HT, Rhoton AL Jr. Microvascular anatomy of the medial temporal region: Part 1: its application to arteriovenous malformation surgery. Neurosurgery. 2010;67(3 Suppl Operative):ons237-76; discussion ons276.
12. Martino J, Vergani F, Robles SG, Duffau H. New insights into the anatomic dissection of the temporal stem with special emphasis on the inferior fronto-occipital fasciculus: implications in surgical approach to left mesiotemporal and temporoinsular structures. Neurosurgery. 2010;66(3 Suppl Operative):4-12.
13. Kucukyuruk B, Richardson RM, Wen HT, Fernandez-Miranda JC, Rhoton AL Jr. Microsurgical anatomy of the temporal lobe and its implications on temporal lobe epilepsy surgery. Epilepsy Res Treat. 2012;2012:769825.
14. Ribas EC, Yagmurlu K, Wen HT, Rhoton AL Jr. Microsurgical anatomy of the inferior limiting insular sulcus and the temporal stem. J Neurosurg. 2015;122(6):1263-73.
15. Wieser HG, Yaşargil MG. Selective amygdalohippocampectomy as a surgical treatment of mesiobasal limbic epilepsy. Surg Neurol. 1982;17(6):445-57.
16. Schramm J, Aliashkevich AF. Temporal mediobasal tumors: a proposal for classification according to surgical anatomy. Acta Neurochir (Wien). 2008;150(9):857-64; discussion 864.
17. Schramm J, Aliashkevich AF. Surgery for temporal mediobasal tumors: experience based on a series of 235 patients. Neurosurgery. 2007;60(2):285-94; discussion 294-5.
18. Tate MC, Kim CY, Chang EF, Polley MY, Berger MS. Assessment of morbidity following resection of cingulate gyrus gliomas. Clinical article. J Neurosurg. 2011;114(3):640-7.

19. Oszvald Á, Quick J, Franz K, Güresir E, Szelényi A, Vatter H, et al. Resection of gliomas in the cingulate gyrus: functional outcome and survival. J Neurooncol. 2012;109(2):341-8.
20. Li H, Ren X, Zhang J, Lin S. Mediobasal and lateral temporal gliomas exhibit different growth patterns, surgical outcomes and prognoses. Clin Neurol Neurosurg. 2015;133:90-5.
21. Mandonnet E, Capelle L, Duffau H. Extension of paralimbic low grade gliomas: toward an anatomical classification based on white matter invasion patterns. J Neurooncol. 2006;78(2):179-85.
22. Duffau H. Resecting diffuse low-grade gliomas to the boundaries of brain functions: a new concept in surgical neuro-oncology. J Neurosurg Sci. 2015;59(4):361-71.
23. Duffau H. Long-term outcomes after supratotal resection of diffuse low grade gliomas: a consecutive series with 11-year follow-up. Acta Neurochir (Wien). 2016;158(1):51-8.
24. Michaud K, Duffau H. Surgery of insular and paralimbic diffuse low-grade gliomas: technical considerations. J Neurooncol. 2016. [Epub ahead of print].
25. Chen XZ, Jiang T, Li SW, Ai L, Dai JP. Dynamic radiological change of gliomas located in the paralimbic system and its clinical significance. Chin Med J Eng. 2008;20;121(8):713-5.
26. Fried I, Kim JH, Spencer DD. Limbic and neocortical gliomas associated with intractable seizures: a distinct clinicopathological group. Neurosurgery. 1994;34(5):815-23; discussion 823-4.
27. Ghareeb F, Duffau H. Intractable epilepsy in paralimbic Word Health Organization Grade II gliomas: should the hippocampus be resected when not invaded by the tumor? J Neurosurg. 2012;116(6):1226-34.
28. MacLean PD. Some psychiatric implications of physiologic studies on frontotemporal portion of the limbic system (visceral brain). Electroencephalogr Clin Neurophysiol. 1952;4:407-18.
29. Yaşargil MG, Krayenbühl N, Roth P, Hsu SP, Yaşargil DC. The selective amygdalohippocampectomy for intractable temporal limbic seizures. J Neurosurg. 2010;112(1):168-85.
30. Marsh JC, Herskovic AM, Gielda BT, Hughes FF, Hoeppner T, Turian J, et al. Intracranial metastatic disease spares the limbic circuit: a review of 697 metastatic lesions in 107 patients. Int J Radiat Oncol Biol Phys. 2010;76(2):504-12.
31. Gozé C, Mansour L, Rigau V, Duffau H. Distinct IDH1/IDH2 mutation profiles in purely insular versus paralimbic WHO Grade II gliomas. J Neurosurg. 2013;118(4):866-72.
32. Tang C, Zhang ZY, Chen LC, Sun Z, Zhang Y, Qin Z, et al. Subgroup characteristics of insular low-grade glioma based on clinical and molecular analysis of 42 cases. J Neurooncol. 2016;126(3): 499-507.
33. Phi JH, Chung CK. Brain tumors in the mesial temporal lobe: long-term oncological outcome. Neurosurg Focus. 2009;27(2):E5.
34. Hori T, Tabuchi S, Kurosaki M, Kondo S, Takenobu A, Watanabe T. Subtemporal amygdalo-hippocampectomy for treating medically intractable temporal lobe epilepsy. Neurosurgery. 1993;33:50-6.
35. Park TS, Bourgeois BF, Silbergeld DL, Dodson WE. Subtemporal transparahippocampal amygdalohippocampectomy for surgical treatment of mesial temporal lobe epilepsy. Technical note. J Neurosurg. 1996;85:1172-6.
36. Russell SM, Kelly PJ. Volumetric stereotaxy and the supratentorial occipitosubtemporal approach in the resection of posterior hippocampus and parahippocampal gyrus lesions. Neurosurgery. 2002;50(5):978-88.
37. Uribe JS, Vale FL. Limited access inferior temporal gyrus approach to mesial basal temporal lobe tumors. J Neurosurg. 2009;110(1):137-46.
38. Türe U, Pamir MN. Small petrosal approach to the middle portion of the mediobasal temporal region: technical case report. Surg Neurol. 2004;61(1):60-7; discussion 67.
39. Sindou MP, Fobé JL. Removal of the roof of the external auditory meatus in approaching the tentorial notch through a low temporal craniotomy. Technical note. J Neurosurg. 1991;74(3):520-2.
40. Smith KA, Spetzler RF. Supratentorial-infraoccipital approach for posteromedial temporal lobe lesions. J Neurosurg. 1995;82(6):940-4.

41. Uchiyama N, Hasegawa M, Kita D, Yamashita J. Paramedian supracerebellar transtentorial approach for a medial tentorial meningioma with supratentorial extension: technical case report. Neurosurgery. 2001;49(6):1470-3; discussion 1473-4.
42. Yonekawa Y, Imhof HG, Taub E, Curcic M, Kaku Y, Roth P, et al. Supracerebellar transtentorial approach to posterior temporomedial structures. J Neurosurg. 2001;94(2):339-45.
43. Moftakhar R, Izci Y, Başkaya MK. Microsurgical anatomy of the supracerebellar transtentorial approach to the posterior mediobasal temporal region: technical considerations with a case illustration. Neurosurgery. 2008;62(3 Suppl 1):1-7; discussion 7-8.
44. Izci Y, Seçkin H, Ateş O, Başkaya MK. Supracerebellar transtentorial transcollateral sulcus approach to the atrium of the lateral ventricle: microsurgical anatomy and surgical technique in cadaveric dissections. Surg Neurol. 2009;72(5):509-14; discussion 514.
45. Türe U, Harput MV, Kaya AH, Baimedi P, Firat Z, Türe H, et al. The paramedian supracerebellar-transtentorial approach to the entire length of the mediobasal temporal region: an anatomical and clinical study. Laboratory investigation. J Neurosurg. 2012;116(4):773-91.
46. Ruban D, Byrne RW, Kanner A, Smith M, Cochran EJ, Roh D, et al. Chronic epilepsy associated with temporal tumors: long-term surgical outcome. Neurosurg Focus. 2009;27(2):E6.
47. Clusmann H, Kral T, Fackeldey E, Blümcke I, Helmstaedter C, von Oertzen J, et al. Lesional mesial temporal lobe epilepsy and limited resections: prognostic factors and outcome. J Neurol Neurosurg Psychiatry. 2004;75(11):1589-96.
48. Von Lehe M, Schramm J. Gliomas of the cingulate gyrus: surgical management and functional outcome. Neurosurg Focus. 2009;27(2):E9.
49. Steiger HJ, Göppert M, Floeth F, Turowski B, Sabel M. Fronto-mesial WHO grade II and III gliomas: specific aspects of tumours arising from the anterior cingulate gyrus. Acta Neurochir (Wien). 2009;151(2):137-40.
50. Talacchi A, Corsini F, Gerosa M. Surgical approaches to tumors of the anterior gyrus cinguli. Neurosurgery. 2010;66(6 Suppl Operative):245-51.
51. Talacchi A, Hasanbelliu A, Fasano T, Gerosa M. Interhemispheric approach to tumors of the posterior gyrus cinguli. Clin Neurol Neurosurg. 2013;115(5):597-602.
52. Vogt BA. Pain and emotion interactions in subregions of the cingulate gyrus. Nat Rev Neurosci. 2005;6:533-44.
53. Davies J, Tawk RG, Lawton MT. The contralateral transcingulate approach: operative technique and results with vascular lesions. Neurosurgery. 2012;71(1 Suppl Operative):4-13; discussion 13-4.

CHAPTER

10 Surgery for Vascular Malformations of the Limbic System

Sahin Hanalioglu, Ilhan Aydin, Hakan Ozalp, Mustafa K Baskaya

INTRODUCTION

Vascular malformations of the central nervous system (CNS) are usually grouped based on their flow characteristics. High flow malformations comprise arteriovenous malformations (AVMs) and arteriovenous fistulas (AVFs). On the other hand, low flow (angiographically occult) malformations include cavernous malformations [CM (cavernous hemangiomas or cavernomas)], capillary telangiectasias and various venous malformations. They can occur anywhere in the CNS including limbic lobe and associated structures. Intricate anatomy of many important interrelated neurovascular structures makes the vascular malformations of the limbic system quite challenging to treat for the neurosurgeons. Nonetheless, extensive anatomical and radiological studies, as well as the developments in surgical techniques and intraoperative tools in recent years, provided remarkable insights into the complex anatomical and functional relationships of the limbic system, which in turn enabled neurosurgeons to excel in the surgical treatment of the lesions involving these regions.

In this chapter, we aim to give an overview of the vascular anatomy of the limbic system, to discuss clinical-radiological features and management options of the vascular malformations of the limbic system with a particular emphasis on surgical approaches and techniques. We concentrated on surgically treatable vascular malformations of the limbic system; namely AVMs and CMs. Therefore, other types of vascular malformations (i.e. capillary telangiectasia, venous malformations) are not covered in this chapter.

AN OVERVIEW OF VASCULAR ANATOMY OF THE LIMBIC SYSTEM

Proper management of vascular malformations of the limbic system requires a thorough understanding of the neural, vascular, cisternal and ventricular anatomy of the limbic system and associated structures (Fig. 10.1). Considering various anatomical classifications of the vascular limbic lesions, here we reviewed related anatomy in two subsections: (1) mediobasal temporal and (2) calloso-cingular (midline interhemispheric) regions.

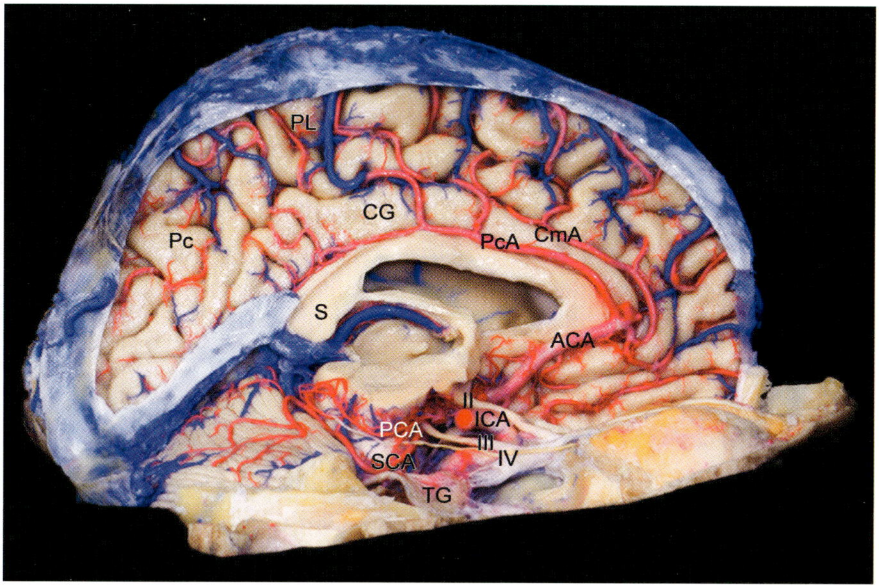

Fig. 10.1: Cadaveric dissection demonstrates limbic and paralimbic structures with neurovascular structures.
(CG: Cingulate gyrus; PL: Paracentral lobule; Pc: Precuneus; S: Splenium; ACA: Anterior cerebral artery; ICA: Internal cerebral artery; PcA: Pericallosal artery; CmA: Callosomarginal artery; PCA: Posterior cerebral artery; SCA: Superior cerebral artery; TG: Trigeminal ganglion; II: Optic nerve; III: Oculomotor nerve; IV: Trochlear nerve).

Mediobasal Temporal Region

The mediobasal temporal region (MTR) is among the most complex anatomical sites in the brain. It contains essential elements of the limbic system such as the amygdala, hippocampus, parahippocampal gyrus, and is surrounded by vital vascular structures.[1,2] De Oliviera and Rhoton divided a medial temporal region into three segments: (1) anterior (from rhinal sulcus to the choroidal point), (2) middle (from the choroidal point to a posterior aspect of the quadrigeminal plate) and (3) posterior (posterior to the quadrigeminal plate).[3,4] Gyral and sulcal anatomy of this region are reviewed in other chapters; therefore, here we will briefly summarize vascular anatomy of this region.

Anterior choroidal artery (AChoA), posterior cerebral artery (PCA) and middle cerebral artery (MCA) provide the main arterial supply to MTR although direct branches from ICA could also contribute partially. The course of the AChoA is of critical importance during surgery in this region. Cisternal and plexal segments of AChoA are divided at the inferior choroidal point where the AChoA enters the temporal horn of the lateral ventricle. Perforating branches arise from late cisternal or early plexal segments of AChoA, commonly referred to as the capsulothalamic artery, which supplies the posterior limb of the internal capsule as well as the tail of the caudate and lateral thalamic nuclei.

Anterior part of the anterior segment of MTR is chiefly irrigated by AChoA (via anterior and posterior uncal arteries, uncohippocampal artery) and MCA (via anterior uncal arteries, unco-parahippocampal arteries) and partially by ICA (via anterior uncal arteries), whereas posterior part of the anterior segment of MTR (posterior entorhinal area) is mainly supplied by PCA (P2a or peduncular segment) (via anterior parahippocampal arteries and anterior hippocampal-parahippocampal arteries). Anastomosis between AChoA and MCA (through anterior uncal arteries) are common. The middle segment of the MTR is exclusively supplied by branches of the PCA (P2p or ambient segment). Anterior and posterior inferior temporal arteries gave off anterior and posterior parahippocampal arteries, respectively. Main arterial supply of the posterior segment of the MTR also comes from PCA branches (P3 and P4 or quadrigeminal segment). Lingual gyrus is irrigated by posteroinferior temporal and calcarine arteries, whereas the isthmus of cingulate gyrus is supplied by the parieto-occipital, splenial, and posterior hippocampal arteries.

The basal vein of Rosenthal (BVR) is the primary venous drainage channel of the MTR. Anterior segment of the MTR is related to the first (striate) portion and the anterior part of the second (peduncular) segment of the BVR, which is created by the union of the deep middle cerebral vein and the inferior striate veins. The common venous drainage patterns of the anterior segment of the MTR are posterior (via the anterior basal anastomotic vein to the posterior peduncular segment of the BVR) (62%) and anterior (via the preuncal vein to the cavernous or sphenoparietal sinuses) (35%). The middle segment of the MTR contains the posterior peduncular (second) and the proximal mesencephalic (third) segments of the BVR. The point where the inferior ventricular vein drains into the anterior peduncular segment of the BVR is where the posterior peduncular segment starts. This point is surgically significant because it corresponds to the border between the anterior and middle segments of the MTR. This junction is also the transition from the crural to ambient cisterns. Posterior drainage via posterior basal anastomotic vein through the vein of Galen complex is the prevailing pattern in the middle MTR. Posterior segment of the MTR is related to distal part of the third or mesencephalic segment of the BVR in the quadrigeminal cistern and empties into the vein of Galen or the internal cerebral vein. The major veins that drain to the posterior segment of the BVR are the lateral mesencephalic, posterior thalamic, posterior longitudinal hippocampal, medial temporal or occipitotemporal cortical and lateral atrial veins.[1,4,5]

Calloso-Cingular Area

Anterior cerebral artery (ACA) is the main arterial supply of the corpus callosum and cingulate gyrus. Both A1 segments join by AComA just before entering into the interhemispheric fissure. Both distal ACAs (A2–5 segments) run upward in front of lamina terminalis. Both distal ACAs make a curve around the genu and then travel backward over the body in the pericallosal cistern. After giving off the cortical branches to medial surface of the hemispheres, the ACA turns around the splenium and ends in the choroid plexus in the roof of the third ventricle. It may anastomose with splenial branches of PCA. The pericallosal artery starts at the anterior communicating artery (AComA) (A2) and courses within the pericallosal sulcus (A2–4), while its largest branch, the callosomarginal artery, courses along the cingulate sulcus and irrigates multiple cortical areas. The origin of callosomarginal artery might be anywhere from just distal to AComA to the level of the genu. The distal ACA gives rise to two types of branches: (1) basal perforators supplying deep structures below the rostrum such as optic chiasm, lamina terminalis, suprachiasmatic area and anterior hypothalamus; (2) cerebral branches with cortical (supplying the cortex and adjacent white matter) and subcortical (to the deep white/gray matter and the corpus callosum) subgroups. The corpus callosum is usually supplied by short callosal arteries arising from the pericallosal artery and penetrating directly into the corpus callosum. These branches not only supply the corpus callosum but also cross through it to irrigate the septum pellucidum, anterior fornix and part of the anterior commissure.[6-10]

The main drainage of the corpus callosum and pericallosal area are via callosal and callosocingulate veins towards the deep venous system of the brain. Typically, they run downward toward the center of the corpus callosum and join to form the subependymal veins, which drain to the septal and the medial atrial veins. Eventually, all these vessels empty into the internal cerebral veins. The basal vein of Rosenthal also receives the deep anterior cerebral vein (posterior orbitofrontal vein), which drains rostral portions of the CC and cingulate gyrus. Furthermore, posterior callosal vein drains the splenium of the corpus callosum and adjacent cerebral surfaces into the great cerebral vein of Galen. The inferior sagittal sinus also receives veins from the adjacent part of the falx, corpus callosum and cingulate gyrus; anterior pericallosal veins being its largest tributaries.[7,8,10-12]

ARTERIOVENOUS MALFORMATIONS

Brain AVMs occur in around 0.1% of the general population representing one-tenth the incidence of intracranial aneurysms. Supratentorial AVMs account for 90% of brain AVMs. Annual hemorrhage risk is about 1–3%, which increases after the first hemorrhage for a year and then decreases to baseline levels. Nearly half of the patients with AVMs present with intracranial hemorrhage (intracerebral, intraventricular and/or subarachnoid) usually between the ages of 10 years and 40 years.[13,14] Ten to thirty percent of the patients have epileptic seizures. While the previous hemorrhage is the most important risk factor for subsequent hemorrhages, presence of associated aneurysms, exclusive deep venous drainage and deep brain location also seem to increase the chance of bleeding.[13-16]

Although many grading scales proved to be successful in predicting surgical morbidity; most of them appeared to be too complex for general use.[16,17] In 1986, Spetzler and Martin proposed a simplified scheme based on size (<3 cm, 3–6 cm, >6 cm), location (eloquent/noneloquent) and venous drainage (deep/superficial), which proved to be very practical and useful.[18] This grading system is currently the most widely used and accepted scheme in the world.

The emergence of microneurosurgery in the 1960s enabled successful treatment of AVMs possible. Advances in surgical techniques and imaging/monitoring technologies along with anatomical knowledge and focused practice in neurovascular surgery dramatically reduced the mortality and morbidity rates while increasing the chances of total removal. In parallel, endovascular treatment options also flourished, and radiosurgery emerged as a third option in the multimodal management of AVMs. Today, these three treatment modalities are used, usually in combination, to successfully treat AVMs of different size, type and locations. The gold standard in the management of AVMs is microsurgical resection with the highest angiographic cure (94–100%) and low morbidity rates (1–10%) in experienced hands. A comprehensive metaanalysis found that while complication rates are similar in three modalities (7.4% for microsurgery, 5.1 for radiosurgery and 6.6% for embolization), complete obliteration rates with microsurgery (96%) are far beyond those of radiosurgery (38%) and embolization (13%).[19]

Based on large-scale studies, many recommendations have been proposed by various authorities regarding the optimal management of brain AVMs. In general, surgical excision is regarded as the primary choice of treatment for Spetzler-Martin grade I and II lesions. However, radiosurgery should also be considered for small lesions, weighing the risks of surgery (due to location or feeding vessel anatomy). For grade III lesions, usually the most heterogeneous group, a multimodality approach with embolization followed by surgery is often feasible. Due to heightened risk of surgery, usually a combination of techniques, starting with embolization, could be considered for Grades IV and V lesions on an individual basis if treatment is deemed necessary.[16,20]

ANATOMICAL CLASSIFICATIONS OF LIMBIC ARTERIOVENOUS MALFORMATIONS

Stein proposed one of the earliest classifications of limbic AVMs in 1984. In a series of 25 medial hemispheric or limbic AVMs (15% of all AVMs), he classified those lesions based on six anatomic regions: (1) Region A: Amygdaloid-uncus region or anteromedial aspect of the temporal lobe; (2) Region B: Parahippocampal and fusiform gyri; (3) Region C: Parapeduncular region or region medial to the trigone (posterior parahippocampal and fusiform gyri); (4) Region D: Splenium and posterior third ventricle; (5) Region E: Corpus callosum-cingulate region; (6) Region F: Septal or medial frontal region.[21]

Yasargil also put a particular emphasis on limbic system AVMs in his large series of surgically treated AVMs in 1988. He classified AVMs into two broad categories; namely convexity (pallial) and central AVMs. In his comprehensive series of 414 surgically treated AVMs, limbic system AVMs comprised a substantial portion of central AVMs (64% of central, 24% of all AVMs). However, as Yasargil noted, it is likely that the actual incidence of central, and therefore limbic, AVM is much lower in general population. He considered amygdalohippocampal (mediobasal temporal) (n = 17), parasplenial (n = 40), cingular (n = 7) and callosal (n = 34) AVMs within the group of limbic AVMs. He further divided mediobasal temporal AVMs into four subgroups: (1) amygdala, (2) anterior, (3) middle and (4) posterior hippocampal. The largest group within limbic AVMs in his series is the parasplenial AVMs, which includes malformations arising in the posterior limbic system where the posterior hippocampus/parahippocampal gyrus connects with the isthmus of the cingulate gyrus.

Arteriovenous malformations of medial/mediobasal temporal lobe are a distinct group of temporal AVMs because of deep location, arterial supply, and venous drainage as well as difficult surgical access due to intervening healthy brain. They are thought to represent about one-fourth of all temporal AVMs in various series.[5,22-24] The literature on pure mediobasal or mesial temporal AVMs is scarce. Most series include temporal AVMs as a whole with varying classifications into subtypes. For example, Rhoton and de Oliveira based their classification on the temporal lobe surfaces: lateral, medial, basal and Sylvian fissure.[4,25] Malik et al. classified them as lateral convexity, mesotemporal and ventricular.[26] Schramm used another classification with temporal lobe, temporomesial, ventricular and Sylvian fissure subtypes.[27] Recently, Lawton and colleagues blended all these classifications into a single practical one with five subtypes: (1) lateral, (2) medial, (3) basal, (4) Sylvian and (5) ventricular.[28] Here, we extracted mediobasal temporal AVMs from the similar series and presented comparative data on clinical features, surgical approaches and outcomes below.

CLINICAL FEATURES OF LIMBIC ARTERIOVENOUS MALFORMATIONS

Drake (1979), Heros (1982) and Stein (1984) presented earliest reports of the surgically treated mesial temporal AVMs. In his series of 25 medial hemispheric or limbic AVMs, Stein reported that these AVMs had clinical features characteristic of AVMs in general. In Yasargil's series, 80% of the patients were under 40 years of age at diagnosis. Various authors reported similar mean ages (30–40 years) for patients with mesial temporal AVMs, which are slightly younger compared with other temporal AVMs. Similarly, a mean age of the patients harboring AVMs of the corpus callosum was found to be 27 ± 13 years in a recent systematic review.

In a few series, mediobasal temporal AVMs present with hemorrhage in the majority of the patients;[28] however in some other series including Yasargil's, seizures were the most common presenting symptom (50–80%).[5,27,29] On the contrary, AVMs in other regions of the limbic system (calloso-cingular, parasplenial) usually present with hemorrhage (80% of the cases).[5,30,31] Interestingly, callosal AVMs have found to cause neuropsychological problems such as memory impairment, lack of insight, impairment in optical-spatial activity, partial "split-brain" syndrome preoperatively. After surgery of anterior CC-AVMs, some patients experienced deterioration of frontal dysfunction, exacerbated disinhibition, lack of insight and impulsivity, while split brain syndrome was encountered after excision of middle and posterior CC-AVMs (with visual neglect).[23,32] Earlier reports lacked a standardized grading scheme for AVMs. However, since the introduction and widespread acceptance of Spetzler-Martin (SM) grading system; most studies have started to report SM grades. In a recent systematic review of CC AVMs, the frequencies of the SM grades were as follows: Grade I (3%), Grade II (28%), Grade III (38%), Grade IV (20%) and Grade V (11%). On the other hand, 80–100% of the reported mediobasal temporal AVMs fall into SM Grades I–III.[27,29,33]

SURGERY OF LIMBIC ARTERIOVENOUS MALFORMATIONS: SURGICAL APPROACHES

Mediobasal Temporal Arteriovenous Malformations

Surgical resection of limbic system AVM is continued to be most challenging surgery in modern neurosurgery. Starting from late 1970s, various authors have reported successful outcomes with varying surgical approaches in these types of AVMs. Today surgery, either alone or with prior embolization, is the mainstay of the management of most AVMs. In one of the earliest comprehensive AVM series, Drake reported on 166 surgically treated AVMs of which six were mesial temporal, and five were corpus callosum AVMs. He used a subtemporal approach to access AVMs in the hippocampal or medial temporal-occipital regions. He underscored the importance of the preservation of vein of Labbe and visual radiations during this approach. Later, Stein and Heros used variations of subtemporal approach in 1980s. Heros combined subtemporal approach with transcortical incisions in the inferior or fusiform gyri to minimize retraction damage.[34] In the same years, Stein published one of the earliest comprehensive studies of medial hemispheric AVMs. Stein utilized an anatomic classification to select the best surgical strategy to attack those AVMs (see above). For region A (amygdala, uncus), Stein preferred pterional craniotomy with transsylvian/transcortical approaches, whereas for region B (parahippocampal/fusiform gyri), subtemporal approach with partial resection of the inferior temporal gyrus was deemed more suitable.[21] In Figures 10.2A to L, a case of ruptured AVM of the dominant fusiform gyrus is demonstrated. In this case, a subtemporal approach was performed with wide sulcal dissection in the middle and inferior temporal sulci (Figs. 10.2A to L).

Yasargil approached the AVMs in the anterior two-thirds of the mediobasal temporal lobe through a pterional craniotomy and transsylvian approach, but for the posterior hippocampal AVMs, he used either a laterobasal or transcortical route (through inferior fusiform gyrus and collateral sulcus). First described by Yasargil for selective amygdalohippocampectomy,[35] the transsylvian-transinsular route has noted advantages of preservation of basal and lateral temporal cortex with limitations including small operative window and associated risk of damage to Meyer's loop due to an entrance to the temporal horn through the roof of the ventricle. Vajkoczy later introduced a transsylvian-transcisternal approach which has overcome the problem of dissection through the ventricular roof and Meyer's loop.[36] However, this approach also comes with drawbacks such as a risk of injury to cisternal structures and a limited operative window. Lawton and colleagues reported favorable results in the surgery of anterior medial temporal AVMs using orbitozygomatic approach, which provided a more anterior trajectory, a shorter working distance to the target and a wider exposure than standard pterional craniotomy.[28,33] For posterior medial and basal temporal AVMs, however, they preferred subtemporal approach through inferior temporal or fusiform gyrus depending on AVM anatomy and the presence of associated hematoma, as did most other authors.

In a comprehensive series of temporal AVMs, Malik et al. also employed transsylvian/transcortical approaches, with the addition of a limited temporal lobectomy (anterior 3 cm) in some cases for anterior MBT AVMs.[26] Ikeda et al. successfully used transcortical/transventricular/transchoroidal fissure approach for a variety of lesions in and around ambient cistern including MBT AVMs.[22] Yasargil also noted that in some complex AVMs with mesial temporal seizures, he performed a partial selective amygdalohippocampectomy to enter the choroidal fissure and ambient cistern aiming to gain early access to the feeders arising from PCA (P2-P3) and distal AChoA. De Oliveira also detailed his surgical techniques complemented with microsurgical anatomical studies in several publications.[3,4,25] Briefly, De Oliveira preferred pretemporal approach (combined pterional and subtemporal approach) with adequate exposure of the temporal pole, for anterior segment MTR AVMs; occipitotemporal sulcus approach, crossing temporal horn and opening the choroidal fissure to reach ambient cistern, for middle

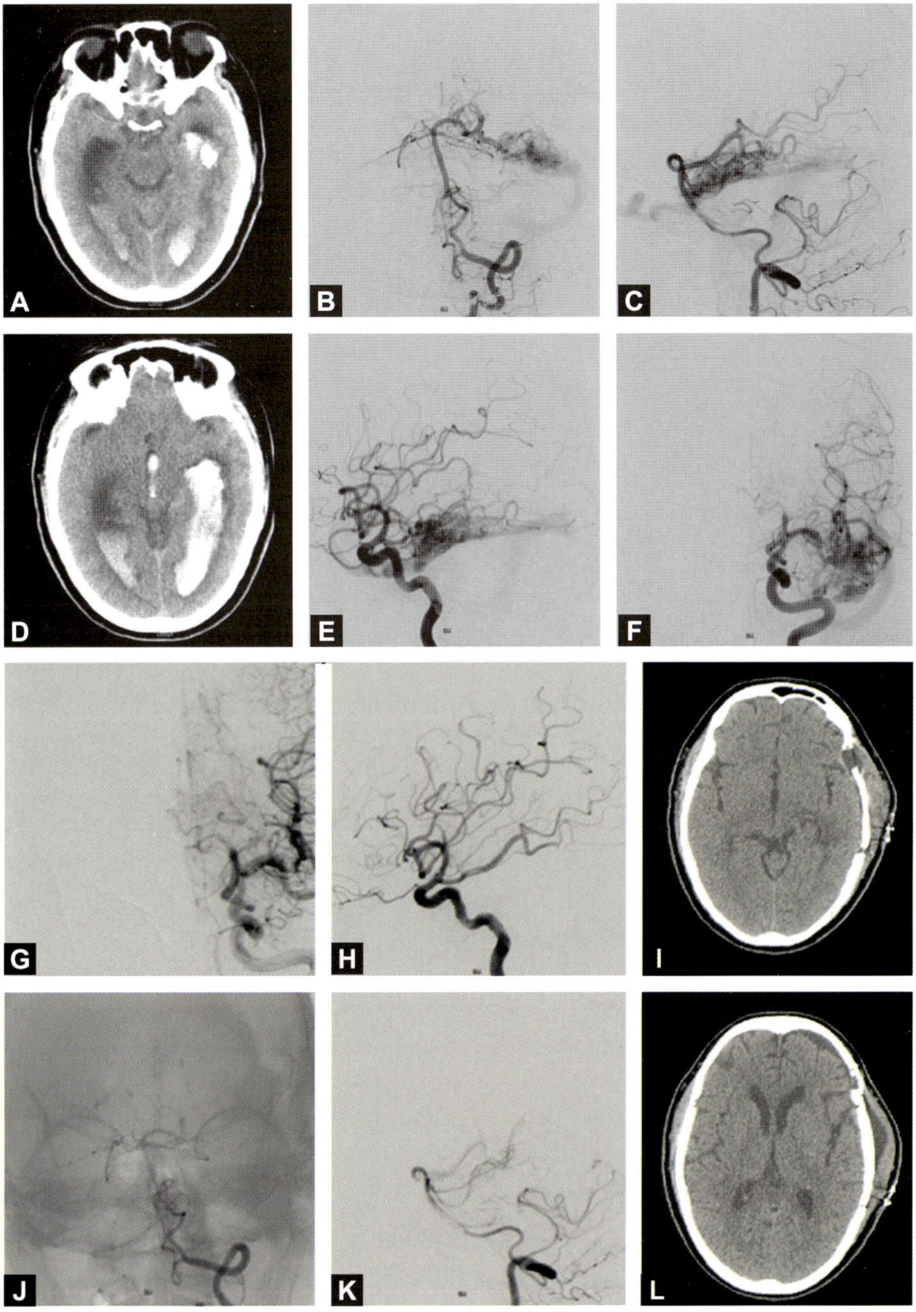

Figs. 10.2A to L: (A and B) A 60-year-old male with known seizures and AVM presented with intraparenchymal and massive intraventricular hemorrhage; (C to F) Bilateral ventriculostomies have been placed. Cerebral angiogram shows large AVM located in the middle segment of the mediobasal temporal region with feeders from the posterior and middle cerebral arteries; (G to J) Postoperative angiogram shows no residual AVM and patent parent arteries and their branches; (K and L) Postoperative late CT scans show postoperative changes and no significant sequelae. The patient made remarkable recovery.

segment MTR AVMs; and posterior (occipital) parafalcine interhemispheric approach through the calcarine and occipitoparietal sulci with minimum retraction of the brain for posterior segment MTR AVMs.[37]

Some authors have thus attempted to combine two or more approaches to gain wider surgical exposure in challenging lesions. One of them was described by Miyamoto et al.[38] They successfully combined subtemporal approach with transventricular/transchoroidal fissure approach to excise various lesions including AVMs in 21 patients. The authors suggested that this combined approach has the advantage of avoiding ischemic complications by allowing direct confirmation of AChoA and thalamoperforating arteries.[38] Some authors recently used supracerebellar transtentorial approach successfully to excise AVMs as well as tumors and cavernomas of the MTR.[25,39]

Parasplenial Arteriovenous Malformations

Yasargil used the term "parasplenial" for AVMs located in the medial basal temporal-parieto-occipital region (other names: incisural, subtrigonal, juxtathalamic, juxtapedincular, posterior parahippocampal, occipitocerebellar-mesencephalic region). He defined this region as the confluence of the hippocampus and isthmus of the cingulate gyrus and fusiform gyrus. He discussed these AVMs as a separate subgroup within limbic AVMs. Although this definition does not directly overlap with a single specific region in the Stein's anatomical classification; it roughly corresponds to Regions C (medial to trigone, parapedincular) and D (splenial, posterior third ventricular region). This area also poses critical challenges to the neurosurgeons. According to Stein, the AVMs in Region C are the most difficult to access. Stein advocated that if the lesion is too large to be exposed by a subtemporal approach with a modest resection of the inferior temporal gyrus, then a transcortical route should be employed or two-stage operation combining posterior infratemporal route with interhemispheric approach should be considered. However, for Region D, he exclusively used posterior interhemispheric parafalx approach which provided safe and adequate exposure. Yasargil excised all parasplenial AVMs through posterior interhemispheric approach, mostly in the sitting position, with the incision in the parasplenial region anterior to P3 and P4. He emphasized that this approach was more adequate than subtemporal or transventricular routes in preserving visual field considering the anatomy of optic radiations.[7]

Calloso-Cingulate Arteriovenous Malformations

Although the surgical management of AVMs of the corpus callosum was reported as early as in the 1950s; first detailed reports of microsurgical technique in relatively larger series were published by Yasargil in 1976.[40,41] He used a small, but elongated parasagittal craniotomy and interhemispheric approach varying in anteroposterior location depending on the exact location of the lesion. Specifically, for anterior and middle callosal AVMs, he used an anterior interhemispheric approach in the supine position while for posterior callosal (splenium) AVMs, the posterior interhemispheric approach in the sitting position was preferable. In giant or multiple callosal AVMs, he either used a combination of anterior and posterior interhemispheric approaches in one session or performed the two-stage operation. Yasargil used the same techniques for operating upon cingulate AVMs. Solomon and Stein also adopted an interhemispheric approach for the lesions of the medial hemispheres, splenium of the corpus callosum, and posterior third ventricle.[21,42] Kim et al. recently described a novel anatomical classification for parafalcine and midline AVMs to aid selection of best surgical strategy. Deriving from a large series of surgically treated AVMs at UCSF (n = 443), authors distributed 132 (30%) midline/parafalcine AVMs into five zones. Superficial-anterior AVMs were approached through anterior interhemispheric route with transcortical dissections in the supine, neutral head position. However, for superficial-middle zone AVMs, the patient is placed supine with the head turned 45° laterally to position AVM side up. With rotating operating table, they achieved to access different aspects (and feeders) of the AVM during the surgery. For superficial-posterior AVMs, they preferred a lateral position with the AVM side up and the head is rotated to position nose down. They used "torcular craniotomy" to expose superior sagittal and transverse sinuses and to open interhemispheric and infraoccipital fissures. Again, by manipulating table rotation, they managed to reach both medial and lateral borders and feeders of the AVM. For deep-anterior AVMs, the patient is placed supine; the head is rotated 90° toward the AVM side, and the neck is angled up 45°. This position allows gravity dependent retraction of the ipsilateral hemisphere and opening of the interhemispheric fissure. We prefer using ipsilateral side down approach for both anterior and middle cingulate AVMs. In Figures 10.3A to J and 10.4A to F, a case of Spetzler-Martin Grade 4 AVM located in the middle cingulate gyrus is demonstrated. In this case, we used interhemispheric approach while the patient was in supine position with almost 70–90° head turn allowing the ipsilateral side falling away from the fissure with gravity. For the deep-posterior lesions, the patient is positioned laterally with the AVM side down, and the head is rotated 45° downward to allow gravity dependent retraction of the occipital lobe and widen the interhemispheric fissure opening. They reported excellent operative results with this classification and tailored surgical strategy. They emphasized the importance of gravity retraction in enhancing operative window for deep midline interhemispheric AVMs.[43,44] Also, a contralateral interhemispheric approach is advocated by some authors for callosal and cingulate lesions including AVMs.[45,46]

Surgical Considerations

A thorough preoperative investigation and careful planning are necessary for AVM surgery. CT is often required to evaluate the hemorrhagic presentation of AVMs. MRI is useful to understand the anatomic location of AVM and its topographic relations with surrounding structures. MR angiography, CT angiography, and the most importantly four-vessel angiography are essential to localize the arterial feeders and drainage veins of the malformation as well as to examine associated aneurysms. MR tractography and functional MRI are helpful in localizing white matter tracts and eloquent cortices, respectively. Preoperative embolization and radiosurgery can be used to downgrade the AVMs in critical locations and therefore to make those lesions more amenable to surgery.[47] Endovascular embolization usually does not achieve complete obliteration but can significantly help to occlude those feeders that are difficult to find and divide early in surgery.[48] The ultimate goal of AVM surgery is complete obliteration. Hence, if an intraoperative or postoperative angiography shows a residual malformation, immediate reoperation should be considered to excise the residual lesion entirely to avoid subsequent

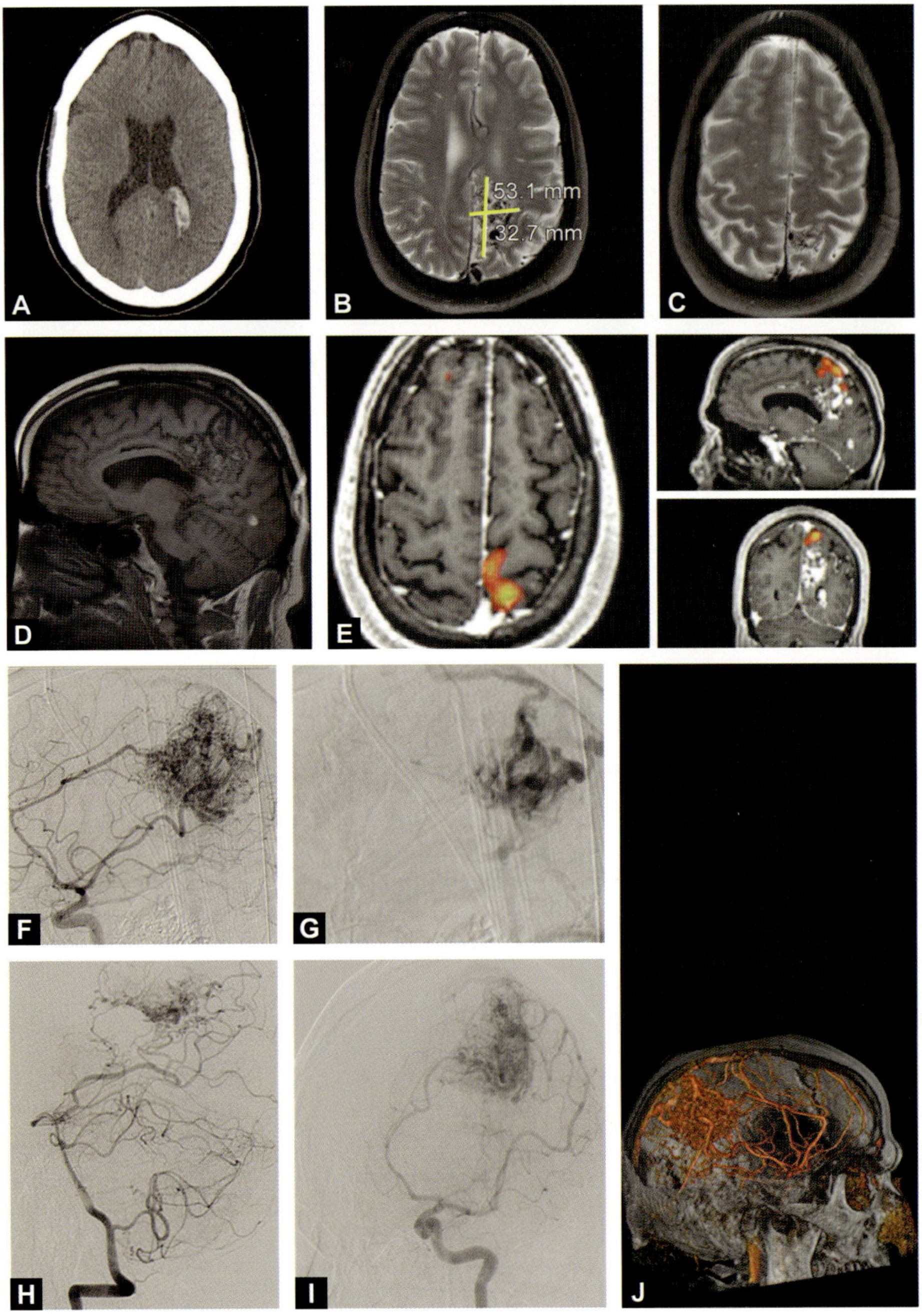

Figs. 10.3A to J: (A) A 45-year-old male with history of multiple intracranial hemorrhages presented with intraventricular hemorrhage; (B to E) T2-axial, T1-sagittal and functional MRIs show large posterior cingulate AVM adjacent to medial aspect of the motor cortex. Note that foot activation adjacent to the AVM in functional MRI; (F to I) Cerebral angiogram shows Spetzler-Martin grade IV AVM with feeders from the anterior, middle and posterior cerebral arteries and drainage into the superficial (sagittal sinus) and deep venous systems; (J) 3D reconstruction image demonstrates all feeders and draining veins.

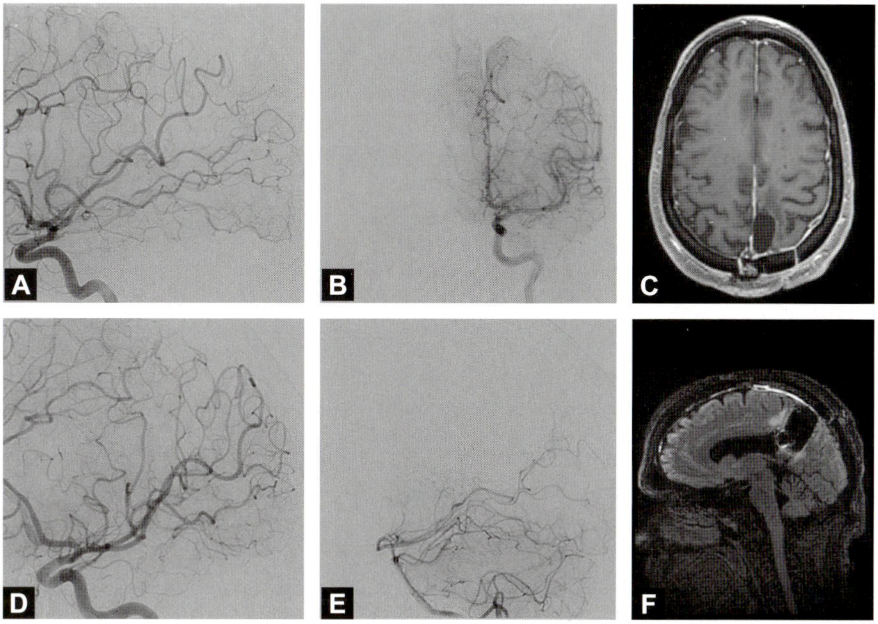

Figs. 10.4A to F: (A to D) Postoperative angiogram shows no residual AVM and preservation of normal vasculature; (E and F) Postoperative late MRIs show extend of resection. The patient made an excellent recovery without any motor or sensory deficits.

hemorrhage. Staged treatment of selected AVMs is also an option to prevent the occurrence of normal perfusion breakthrough and to achieve satisfactory obliteration of selected AVMs with multiple complex arterial feeders, associated aneurysms or dural component.[49]

The fundamental principle of AVM surgery is to find and coagulate arterial feeders first, and then circumscribe the malformation (nidus) and to coagulate and divide main drainage vein(s) at the end. It is essential to preserve the main venous drainage until very last to prevent the AVM from swelling and producing spontaneous hemorrhage.[10] While selecting the surgical approach, one should take into account the exact position of arterial feeders and the structures to be traversed along the surgical route. The goal is to resect the AVM without interfering with normal parenchyma and its vascular supply. Meticulous attention to the microneurosurgical techniques is imperative to a successful surgical outcome. Arterial feeders should be identified correctly and divided step by step. En passage arteries are of particular importance in AVM surgery and must be preserved to avoid functional deficits. Circumferential dissection of the nidus should follow the surrounding gliotic tissue. Once, the arterial supply is obliterated, and the lesion is completely dissected from the parenchyma, the main drainage vein should be coagulated and cut as the final step of the surgery.

In the anterior approaches to the mediobasal temporal AVMs, an extensive Sylvian fissure opening is required. Once the medial surface of the AVM is accessed, the feeding arteries originating from AChoA and PCA should be identified and divided. When the lesion is dissected circumferentially, the feeding arteries from the lateral margin, usually through ventricle, also deserve special attention. It should be noted that basal vein of Rosenthal is not seen until the end of the dissection and care should be taken to distinguish it from a feeding artery. Before reaching this deep draining vein, superficial drainage veins should be coagulated as the dissection deepens and the lesion darkens.[33] The subtemporal approach used for more posteriorly located MBT AVMs also allows early exposure of the arterial feeders from the medial surface of the AVM. Although this approach avoids damage to optic radiations, it carries a risk of excessive retraction of the temporal lobe and injury to the vein of Labbe. Therefore, various authors added either a transcortical incision or modest resection through inferior portion of the temporal lobe to minimize these risks.[34]

For parasplenial AVMs, Yasargil put a particular emphasis on venous anatomy, including basal, internal occipital and mesencephalic veins, which may complicate surgical dissection. Yasargil, therefore, used a posterior interhemispheric approach by making an incision in the parasplenial region anterior to P3 and P4 segments.[7]

The interhemispheric approach is the standard surgical route for most callosal AVMs. It is important to extend craniotomy a few millimeters across the midline. Great care is needed not to tear any bridging veins. Usually, 2–3 cm of cortical margin free of bridging veins provides a sufficiently broad operative window. It is important, albeit challenging, to preserve cortical draining veins until the end of the procedure if they are the main draining channels of the AVM. Once the AVM is exposed, the arterial feeders from anterior pericallosal arteries on the side of larger lateral extension should be occluded first. Dissection through the corpus callosum should be started on the usual side of the corpus callosum (away from AVM) and as far away from the main venous drainage as possible, i.e. from anterior for anterior CC-AVMs, but from posterior for middle CC-AVMs because of the position of the septal vein. Once the ventricle is entered, dissection of the abnormal side of the corpus callosum can be performed taking care of the draining septal vein. To preserve thalamostriatal and internal cerebral veins are of utmost importance during dissection in this region. For posterior callosal or splenial AVMs, upon sufficient craniotomy crossing midline and extending to transverse sinus, occipital lobe is retracted laterally to expose the callosal and quadrigeminal cisterns anterior and inferior to the falcotentorial junction. The bluish appearance of the quadrigeminal cistern could be confused with a large vein. Thick and opaque arachnoid bands over the cistern should be dissected carefully. Following the arachnoid opening, splenium, vein of Galen, ambient and quadrigeminal cisterns and their vascular content should be clearly visualized. Then the AVM could be resected first with the elimination of the arterial supply from anterior and posterior pericallosal feeders and occasionally from parieto-occipital and/or calcarine branches of PCA. After that, the nidus is dissected circumferentially, and finally, the main draining vein to the medial atrial vein is identified and divided. Sometimes, a partial resection of posterior fusiform and cingulate gyri could be needed to remove the lesion completely. The same surgical principles apply for cingulate AVMs. Nevertheless, the main problem in these lesions is often the extraordinary depth of the cingulate sulcus in interhemispheric approach and great care, therefore, is needed during dissection of it. Also, dual major venous drainage to both superficial (to the convexity via the medial hemisphere) and deep (to the vein of Galen) veins may complicate the resection of cingulate AVMs.[7,21,50]

Surgical Outcomes

Multimodality approach, proper surgical planning, intraoperative guidance with imaging tools, detailed anatomical knowledge and rigorous training and experience in microsurgery have yielded satisfying results in the surgery of limbic AVMs in the past decades. Neurosurgical giants such as Drake, Yasargil, Heros and Stein paved the way for successful resection of these once inoperable lesions with minimal or no injury to the normal vasculature and parenchyma.

Some studies have focused on the clinical outcomes of temporal AVMs. Few of them detailed the data about medial or mediobasal subgroup. Most of the published literature presents gratifying results with surgical management of temporal AVMs (mortality 0–5%, permanent morbidity 5–25%). Complete obliteration rates are above 90%. Yasargil reported good operative results in 95% of the patients. Ninety one percent of the patients had no preoperative visual field defects (VFD) postoperatively. Worsening of the visual field occurred in only 6% of surgically treated temporal AVMs in his series.[7] Malik et al. reported 25% of the patients with temporal AVMs had surgical morbidity lasting more than 3 months. Nonetheless, this figure dropped to 13% when isolated field deficits were excluded.[26] Schramm's group reported higher rates of surgical morbidity, particularly hemiparesis (25%), in mesial temporal AVMs. However, although vision could be affected in an early postoperative period, their data indicate that significant visual field defect caused by the surgery is not very common (2.7% permanent disabling VFD after surgery).[27] Lawton and colleagues also had satisfying clinical outcomes with no mortality but 11% and 31% transient surgical morbidity in basal and medial temporal AVMs, respectively. A recent study exploring visual field defects and epilepsy outcomes after the surgery of temporal AVMs found that 24% patients showed new VFDs, but 84% of the patients had preservation of full visual fields at long-term follow-up.[29] Epilepsy control is also an important component of the AVM management and successful surgery accomplishes seizure control rates as high as 85–90% in the temporal AVMs.[7,12,29]

Yasargil achieved satisfying operative results for the parasplenial AVMs (85% good, 12.5% moderate and 2.5% death). For callosal AVMs, he accomplished good operative results in 95.6% of those without preoperative deficits, whereas in 72.7% of those with preoperative deficits. Kim et al. reported similar figures (86% good outcomes) in parafalcine and midline AVMs. In their series, 56% of the patients neurologically improved while 31% remained unchanged. Transient new neurological deficits were observed in 16.6% of the patients, but all of them resolved by late follow-up. Surgical mortality rate was 3%.[51,52] A recent systematic review showed that microsurgical management yielded complete obliteration rate of 94% in callosal AVMs, however, 32% of the patients developed permanent complications after the surgery.[31]

CAVERNOUS MALFORMATIONS

The majority of CMs occur in a supratentorial compartment (within white matter associated with rolandic and temporal areas), although brainstem and cerebellar cavernomas constitute 25% of all CMs.[53,54] Some large-scale natural history studies have reported various symptomatic hemorrhage rates ranging from 0.1 to 2.7% per lesion-year and 0.7–6% per patient-year. Recent large cohort data suggested that 5-year risk of the first hemorrhage is 2.4%, and 5-year risk of seizure without prior hemorrhage or neurological deficits is around 4%. Prior hemorrhage raises the risk of recurrent hemorrhage substantially (5-year risk: 29%).[55,56] Previous hemorrhage, deep/infratentorial location and female sex have been shown to increase the risk of bleeding.[54]

Management options for CMs include observation for asymptomatic ones, while some neurosurgeons advocate for the removal of solitary, easily accessible lesions in noneloquent areas even if asymptomatic. Radiosurgery is another option for deep-seated, poorly accessible CMs. However, its role in the control of hemorrhage and enlargement of CM is not well established.[57] Radiologically proven enlargement of the lesion, progressive neurologic deficits or repeated hemorrhages with neurologic impairment require surgical removal of the CMs. Deep-seated CMs (brainstem, basal ganglia, thalamus, etc.) or those situated in the eloquent cortices are particularly challenging for neurosurgeons to excise without damage to normal neural tissue and require special expertise in the field. Although microsurgery achieves excellent seizure control rates (up to 80%) as well, seizures alone that are controlled with medication do not constitute an indication for surgery unless there is a high risk of bleeding or above-mentioned reasons to operate.

LIMBIC CAVERNOUS MALFORMATIONS: ANATOMIC DISTRIBUTION AND CLINICAL FEATURES

Literature regarding the CMs located specifically in the limbic system is scarce possibly due to the predilection of CMs to other areas of the brain. Particular emphasis has been placed on the surgery of the brainstem CMs in the literature because of their relatively higher incidence and difficulties in their management. However, temporal CMs are also frequent (15–20%) and recently gained attention due to their association with refractory epilepsy.[58-61] Therefore, one can assume that mesial temporal CMs are probably the most common of the (surgically treated) limbic CMs although there are no exact figures about their incidences or relative frequencies. In Yasargil's series of 28 surgically treated cavernomas; two had amygdalohippocampal CMs (in addition to four temporal CMs), and one had parasplenial CM.[5] Nevertheless, he mentions 12 cavernomas among 132 mediobasal temporal tumors (9%), and two cavernomas among 54 cingulate tumors (4%) later in his chapter on limbic and paralimbic tumors.[62] Since no study grouped limbic CMs separately thus far, we tried to extract them from different series published in the literature. Based on the numbers provided by authors, all pure limbic CMs likely account for less than 10% of all surgically treated CMs. Mediobasal temporal CMs are relatively more common than those in the other parts of the limbic system. In Helsinki group's extensive series of 360 CMs, 15% were temporal, but not an exact figure was given regarding the limbic (mediobasal) subgroup.[43] In the series of large-volume epilepsy surgery centers, however, mediobasal temporal CMs may constitute up to 10% of all epilepsy surgery cases, and 10–20% of all cerebral CMs.[43,59,63-65] Clear descriptions regarding the exact anatomical location and seizure semiology lack in the published literature.[59] CMs in the other regions of the limbic system are rare. Only small series and individual case reports exist about the clinical characteristics and surgical management of the CMs located in the corpus callosum, cingulate gyrus, parasplenial area and associated limbic structures.[46,57,66-68]

Mediobasal temporal CMs were almost exclusively present with seizures, complex partial seizures being the most common form. Drug-resistant or chronic epilepsy, which occurs in up to 40% of cerebral CMs, is usually the main reason for treatment of those lesions.[59] Published reports often include them within the epilepsy surgery cohorts. In the series of Bonn group, mediobasal temporal CMs account for 29% of drug-resistant epilepsy associated with CMs. A hemorrhagic presentation is less frequent in those lesions compared with other parts of the limbic system or CNS.[59]

SURGERY OF LIMBIC CAVERNOUS MALFORMATIONS

Surgical Approaches and Techniques

The main reasons for surgery of mediobasal temporal CMs are to eliminate hemorrhage risk and to control associated epilepsy. Most authors strongly recommend early timing of the resection for the better control of epilepsy.[59,69] The general principles of CMs surgery follow those of tumors in the MTR. Nevertheless, their well-circumscribed nature within a gliotic plane makes their surgical resection relatively easier and safer. Also, the control of bleeding is not very difficult due to the low-flow characteristics and the absence of the main arterial supplies.[30,70] Small transsulcal or transcortical incision is sufficient to reach and circumscribe the lesion from surrounding gliotic tissue. Transit vessels and most importantly venous anomalies should be carefully identified and preserved during the cavernoma surgery.

Many approaches, mentioned earlier for limbic tumors and AVMs, are also applicable for CMs located within limbic areas. The experience in this field greatly benefited from epilepsy and AVM surgeries.[30] In general, variations of anterior transsylvian (with either standard pterional or orbitozygomatic craniotomies) approaches can be used to excise medial temporal CMs. Some authors have preferred epilepsy surgery approaches (i.e. anterior temporal lobectomy, amygdalohippocampectomy) to resect adjacent mesial temporal structures in addition to cavernoma. The rationale behind this strategy is threefold: (1) hemosiderin rim around cavernoma is possibly epileptogenic; (2) most patients with mediobasal temporal CMs also have some degree of mesial temporal sclerosis; (3) pre- and intraoperative electrophysiological studies usually show epileptogenic zones wider than cavernoma itself.[59,65] Thus, a detailed presurgical epileptologic workup including MRI, video EEG and sometimes invasive monitoring is strongly recommended by various authors.[59] Also, intraoperative electrocorticography is deemed necessary for guiding tailored resections by most epilepsy surgeons.[64] Neuronavigation and intraoperative MRI also seem to increase the accuracy of resections and improve the surgical results regarding epilepsy control.[71]

Regarding more posteriorly located CMs of the MTR, posterior approaches, in contrast to subtemporal and transcortical routes, have been gaining popularity among neurosurgeons nowadays. Recently, modifications of supracerebellar transtentorial approach have been introduced by various authors to successfully remove some posterior mediobasal temporal lobe lesions including CMs.[25,39,72,73] This approach is particularly useful for pathologies in the dominant temporal lobe because it avoids the retraction of eloquent cortex, the vein of Labbe and transcortical incisions. On the other hand, lesions in the middle portion of medial temporal lobe are considered as the most difficult ones to access. Anterior (e.g. transsylvian/transinsular, transsylvian/transcisternal, transsylvian/translimen insula, temporal lobectomy), lateral (subtemporal approaches with or without transcortical incisions/resections, small petrosal approach) and posterior approaches (supracerebellar transtentorial and occipital interhemispheric) provide certain degrees of exposure to the middle portion with their own limitations. (Figs. 10.5A to I).[2,51,74] Therefore, careful presurgical examination of imaging data, a detailed anatomical study of the region and surgeon's experience should be taken into consideration while selecting the best surgical strategy to attack those lesions. Some large CMs and those involving more than one region of the MTR or extending toward posteriorly to the isthmus of the cingulate often require combined approaches or staged operations.

In some instances and selected cases, even minimally invasive approaches could be used to remove CMs safely in respective regions. Using minimally invasive supraorbital subfrontal keyhole approach Reisch et al. achieved complete removal of 14 out of 21 dominant mediobasal temporal lesions including two CMs. Recently, Ding et al. used a minimally invasive endoport system to remove three deep-seated CMs via small cranial and dural openings.[75]

For midline interhemispheric CMs, anterior or posterior interhemispheric approaches are classically used with slight variations depending on the exact location of the lesion. On the other hand, Lawton and colleagues advocated for contralateral transcallosal or transcingulate approaches for a variety of lesions located in the calloso-cingular area.[33,76] Surgical approaches were detailed above in the section of AVM surgery.

Surgical Outcomes

With the advent of radiological imaging and surgical techniques, mortality and morbidity rates of cavernoma surgery also diminished significantly. Surgical morbidity following the surgery of mediobasal temporal CMs includes transient neurological deficits, chiefly visual defects, language problems and hemiparesis, which substantially resolve during the follow-up. Persistent postoperative deficits are between 5% and 10% in different series.[59]

Seizure outcomes depend on several factors. One of the well-established factors is the duration of seizures preoperatively. Although seizure control is generally quite satisfying in CM-associated epilepsy as a whole (70–90%); the patients with single/few or short duration of seizures have better seizure control rates (85–100%) as compared with drug-resistant epilepsy or longer duration of epilepsy (70–80%).[59-61] Another factor is the extent of resection in medial temporal CMs. Many authors advocate for hemosiderin rim removal in addition to lesionectomy due to its possible epileptogenic effects. Some groups reported better results with this strategy,[77,78] whereas others favored pure lesionectomy to avoid complications.[61] Recently tailored approaches and extended resections for selected cases have been adopted by some authors based on careful preoperative evaluation and intraoperative electrocorticographic recordings. Extending the resection to include anteromedial temporal structures offered better seizure control rates in the long-term follow-up in most recent studies.[59,60,78-80] Overall, the surgical results of CM-associated mesial temporal lobe epilepsy (MTLE) are regarded superior to those of hippocampal sclerosis associated MTLE.[81]

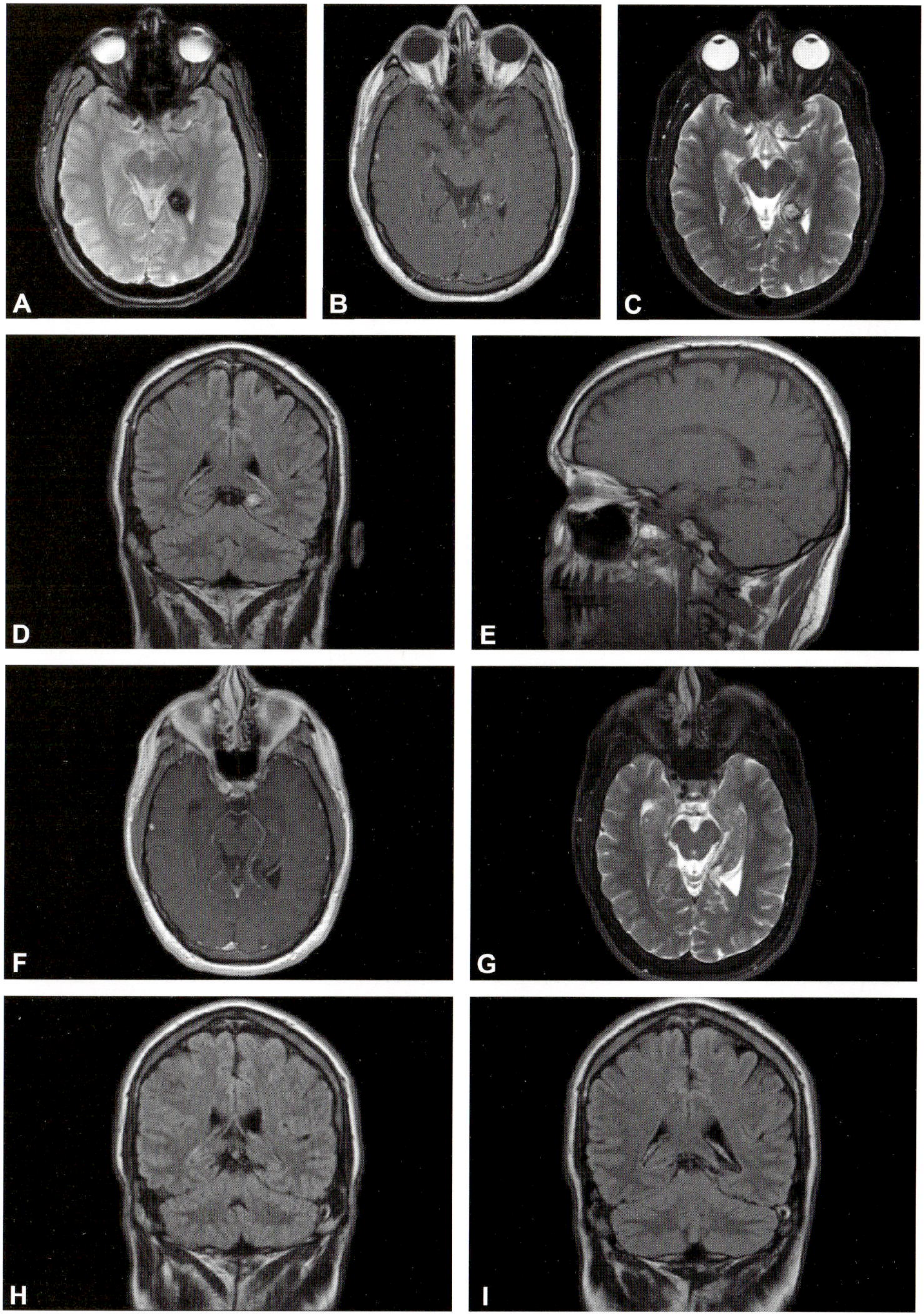

Figs. 10.5A to I: Preoperative MRIs of a 48-year-old patient who presented with partial seizures. (A to E) MRIs show a hemorrhagic lesion located in the posterior parahippocampal gyrus; (F to I) Postoperative MRIs show gross total resection of cavernous malformation. The patient made an excellent recovery and has been seizure free since surgery.

REFERENCES

1. Wen HT, Rhoton AL Jr, de Oliveira E, Cardoso AC, Tedeschi H, Baccanelli M, et al. Microsurgical anatomy of the temporal lobe: part 1: mesial temporal lobe anatomy and its vascular relationships as applied to amygdalohippocampectomy. Neurosurgery. 1999;45(3):549-91; discussion 591-2.
2. Campero A, Tróccoli G, Martins C, Fernandez-Miranda JC, Yasuda A, Rhoton AL Jr. Microsurgical approaches to the medial temporal region: an anatomical study. Neurosurgery. 2006;59 (4 Suppl 2): ONS279-307; discussion ONS307-8.
3. de Oliveira E, Tedeschi H, Siqueira MG, Ono M, Rhoton AL Jr, Peace D. Anatomic principles of cerebrovascular surgery for arteriovenous malformations. Clin Neurosurg. 1994;41:364-80.
4. Fernández-Miranda JC, de Oliveira E, Rubino PA, Wen HT, Rhoton AL Jr. Microvascular anatomy of the medial temporal region: part 1: its application to arteriovenous malformation surgery. Neurosurgery. 2010;67(3 Suppl Operative):ons237-76; discussion ons276.
5. Yaşargil MG. Microneurosurgery IIIB: AVM of the brain, clinical considerations, general and special operative techniques, surgical results, nonoperated cases, cavernous and venous angiomas, neuroanesthesia. New York: Georg Thieme Verlag; 1988.
6. Perlmutter D, Rhoton AL Jr. Microsurgical anatomy of the distal anterior cerebral artery. J Neurosurg. 1978;49(2):204-28.
7. Yaşargil MG. Microneurosurgery IIIA: AVM of the brain, history, embryology, pathological considerations, hemodynamics, diagnostic studies, microsurgical anatomy. New York: Georg Thieme Verlag; 1987.
8. Da Pian R, Pasqualin A, Scienza R, Cappelletto B, Licata C. Surgical Experience with Callosal-Cingular and Inferior Limbic AVMs. In: Da Pian R, Pasqualin A (Eds). New Trends in Management of Cerebro-Vascular Malformations. Verona, Italy: Springer; 1994. pp. 399-409.
9. Rhoton AL Jr. The cerebral veins. Neurosurgery. 2002;51(Suppl 1):S159-S205.
10. Yaşargil MG, Türe U, Yaşargil DC. Surgical anatomy of supratentorial midline lesions. Neurosurg Focus. 2005;18(6B):E1.
11. Wolfram-Gabel R, Maillot C. The venous vascularization of the corpus callosum in man. Surg Radiol Anat. 1992;14(1):17-21.
12. Rhoton AL Jr. The supratentorial arteries. Neurosurgery. 2002;51(Suppl 1):S53-S120.
13. Fleetwood IG, Steinberg GK. Arteriovenous malformations. Lancet. 2002;359(9309):863-73.
14. Choi JH, Mohr JP. Brain arteriovenous malformations in adults. Lancet Neurol. 2005;4(5):299-308.
15. Al-Shahi R, Warlow C. A systematic review of the frequency and prognosis of arteriovenous malformations of the brain in adults. Brain. 2001;124(Pt 10):1900-26.
16. Spagnuolo E. Surgical management of cerebral arteriovenous malformations. In: Quinones-Hinojosa A (Ed). Schmidek and Sweet Operative Neurosurgical Techniques, 6th edition. Philadelphia, PA: Elsevier Saunders; 2012. Chapter 83.
17. Luessenhop AJ, Gennarelli TA. Anatomical grading of supratentorial arteriovenous malformations for determining operability. Neurosurgery. 1977;1(1):30-5.
18. Spetzler RF, Martin NA. A proposed grading system for arteriovenous malformations. J Neurosurg. 1986;65(4):476-83.
19. van Beijnum J, van der Worp HB, Buis DR, Al-Shahi Salman R, Kappelle LJ, Rinkel GJ, et al. Treatment of brain arteriovenous malformations: a systematic review and meta-analysis. JAMA. 2011;306(18):2011-9.
20. Ogilvy CS, Stieg PE, Awad I, Brown RD Jr, Kondziolka D, Rosenwasser R, et al. AHA Scientific Statement: Recommendations for the management of intracranial arteriovenous malformations: a statement for healthcare professionals from a special writing group of the Stroke Council, American Stroke Association. Stroke. 2001;32(6):1458-71.
21. Stein BM. Arteriovenous malformations of the medial cerebral hemisphere and the limbic system. J Neurosurg. 1984;60(1):23-31.

22. Ikeda K, Shoin K, Mohri M, Kijima T, Someya S, Yamashita J. Surgical indications and microsurgical anatomy of the transchoroidal fissure approach for lesions in and around the ambient cistern. Neurosurgery. 2002;50(5):1114-9; discussion 1120.
23. Buklina SB. The unilateral spatial neglect phenomenon in patients with arteriovenous malformations of deep brain structures. Neurosci Behav Physiol. 2002;32(6):555-60.
24. Martin NA, Wilson CB. Medial occipital arteriovenous malformations. Surgical treatment. J Neurosurg. 1982;56(6):798-802.
25. de Oliveira JG, Párraga RG, Chaddad-Neto F, Ribas GC, de Oliveira EP. Supracerebellar transtentorial approach-resection of the tentorium instead of an opening—to provide broad exposure of the mediobasal temporal lobe: anatomical aspects and surgical applications: clinical article. J Neurosurg. 2012;116(4):764-72.
26. Malik GM, Seyfried DM, Morgan JK. Temporal lobe arteriovenous malformations: surgical management and outcome. Surg Neurol. 1996;46(2):106-14; discussion 114-5.
27. Boström A, Schaller K, Seifert J, Schramm J. The place for surgical treatment for AVM involving the temporal lobe. Acta Neurochir (Wien). 2011;153(2):271-8.
28. Gabarrós Canals A, Rodríguez-Hernández A, Young WL, Lawton MT. UCSF Brain AVM Study Project. Temporal lobe arteriovenous malformations: anatomical subtypes, surgical strategy, and outcomes. J Neurosurg. 2013;119(3):616-28.
29. Lopez-Ojeda P, Labib M, Burneo J, Lownie SP. Temporal lobe arteriovenous malformations: surgical outcomes with a focus on visual field defects and epilepsy. Neurosurgery. 2013;73(5):854-62; discussion 862; quiz 862.
30. Yaşargil MG, Krayenbühl N, Roth P, Hsu SP, Yaşargil DC. The selective amygdalohippocampectomy for intractable temporal limbic seizures. J Neurosurg. 2010;112(1):168-85.
31. Pabaney AH, Ali R, Kole M, Malik GM. Arteriovenous malformations of the corpus callosum: Pooled analysis and systematic review of literature. Surg Neurol Int. 2016;7(Suppl 9):S228-36.
32. Buklina SB. The corpus callosum, interhemisphere interactions, and the function of the right hemisphere of the brain. Neurosci Behav Physiol. 2005;35(5):473-80.
33. Du R, Young WL, Lawton MT. "Tangential" resection of medial temporal lobe arteriovenous malformations with the orbitozygomatic approach. Neurosurgery. 2004;54(3):645-51; discussion 651-2.
34. Heros RC. Arteriovenous malformations of the medial temporal lobe. Surgical approach and neuroradiological characterization. J Neurosurg. 1982;56(1):44-52.
35. Yaşargil MG, Teddy PJ, Roth P. Selective amygdalo-hippocampectomy. Operative anatomy and surgical technique. Adv Tech Stand Neurosurg. 1985;12:93-123.
36. Vajkoczy P, Krakow K, Stodieck S, Pohlmann-Eden B, Schmiedek P. Modified approach for the selective treatment of temporal lobe epilepsy: transsylvian-transcisternal mesial en bloc resection. J Neurosurg. 1998;88(5):855-62.
37. Wang H, Zhang R, Yu W, Zhong P, Tan D. The posterior subtemporal keyhole approach combined with the transchoroidal approach to the ambient cistern: microsurgical anatomy and image-guided quantitative analysis. Acta Neurochir (Wien). 2010;152(11):1933-42.
38. Miyamoto S, Kataoka H, Ikeda A, Takahashi J, Usui K, Takayama M, et al. A combined subtemporal and transventricular/transchoroidal fissure approach to medial temporal lesions. Neurosurgery. 2004;54(5):1162-7; discussion 1167-9.
39. Swanson KI, Cikla U, Uluc K, Baskaya MK. Supracerebellar transtentorial approach to the tentorial incisura and beyond. Neurosurg Focus. 2016;40(Video Suppl 1):2016.1.FocusVid.15444.
40. Yasargil MG, Jain KK, Antic J, Laciga R, Kletter G. Arteriovenous malformations of the anterior and the middle portions of the corpus callosum: microsurgical treatment. Surg Neurol. 1976;5(2):67-80.
41. Yaşargil MG, Jain KK, Antic J, Laciga R. Arteriovenous malformations of the splenium of the corpus callosum: microsurgical treatment. Surg Neurol. 1976;5(1):5-14.
42. Solomon RA, Stein BM. Surgical management of arteriovenous malformations that follow the tentorial ring. Neurosurgery. 1986;18(6):708-15.

43. Kivelev J, Niemelä M, Blomstedt G, Roivainen R, Lehecka M, Hernesniemi J. Microsurgical treatment of temporal lobe cavernomas. Acta Neurochir (Wien). 2011;153(2):261-70.
44. Chi JH, Lawton MT. Posterior interhemispheric approach: surgical technique, application to vascular lesions, and benefits of gravity retraction. Neurosurgery. 2006;59(1 Suppl 1):ONS41-9; discussion ONS41-9.
45. Machado de Almeida G, Shibata MK, Nakagawa EJ. Contralateral parafalcine approach for parasagittal and callosal arteriovenous malformations. Neurosurgery. 1984;14(6):744-6.
46. Davies J, Tawk RG, Lawton MT. The contralateral transcingulate approach: operative technique and results with vascular lesions. Neurosurgery. 2012;71(1 Suppl Operative):4-13; discussion 13-4.
47. Abla AA, Rutledge WC, Seymour ZA, Guo D, Kim H, Gupta N, et al. A treatment paradigm for high-grade brain arteriovenous malformations: volume-staged radiosurgical downgrading followed by microsurgical resection. J Neurosurg. 2015;122(2):419-32.
48. Başkaya MK, Heros RC. Indications for and complications of embolization of cerebral arteriovenous malformations. J Neurosurg. 2006;104(2):183-6; discussion 186-7.
49. Andrews BT, Wilson CB. Staged treatment of arteriovenous malformations of the brain. Neurosurgery. 1987;21(3):314-23.
50. Reisch R, Stadie A, Kockro R, Gawish I, Schwandt E, Hopf N. The minimally invasive supraorbital subfrontal key-hole approach for surgical treatment of temporomesial lesions of the dominant hemisphere. Minim Invasive Neurosurg. 2009;52(4):163-9.
51. Straus D, Byrne RW, Sani S, Serici A, Moftakhar R. Microsurgical anatomy of the transsylvian translimen insula approach to the mediobasal temporal lobe: Technical considerations and case illustration. Surg Neurol Int. 2013;4:159.
52. Kim YB, Young WL, Lawton MT; UCSF BAVM Study Project. Parafalcine and midline arteriovenous malformations: surgical strategy, techniques, and outcomes. J Neurosurg. 2011;114(4):984-93.
53. Voigt K, Yaşargil MG. Cerebral cavernous haemangiomas or cavernomas. Incidence, pathology, localization, diagnosis, clinical features and treatment. Review of the literature and report of an unusual case. Neurochirurgia (Stuttg). 1976;19(2):59-68.
54. Washington CW, McCoy KE, Zipfel GJ. Update on the natural history of cavernous malformations and factors predicting aggressive clinical presentation. Neurosurg Focus. 2010;29(3):E7.
55. Al-Shahi Salman R, Hall JM, Horne MA, Moultrie F, Josephson CB, Bhattacharya JJ, et al. Untreated clinical course of cerebral cavernous malformations: a prospective, population-based cohort study. Lancet Neurol. 2012;11(3):217-24.
56. Al-Shahi Salman R. The outlook for adults with epileptic seizure(s) associated with cerebral cavernous malformations or arteriovenous malformations. Epilepsia. 2012;53(Suppl 4):34-42.
57. Chang EF, Gabriel RA, Potts MB, Berger MS, Lawton MT. Supratentorial cavernous malformations in eloquent and deep locations: surgical approaches and outcomes. Clinical article. J Neurosurg. 2011;114(3):814-27.
58. Shan YZ, Fan XT, Meng L, An Y, Xu JK, Zhao GG. Treatment and outcome of epileptogenic temporal cavernous malformations. Chin Med J (Engl). 2015;128(7):909-13.
59. von der Brelie C, Malter MP, Niehusmann P, Elger CE, von Lehe M, Schramm J. Surgical management and long-term seizure outcome after epilepsy surgery for different types of epilepsy associated with cerebral cavernous malformations. Epilepsia. 2013;54(9):1699-706.
60. Yeon JY, Kim JS, Choi SJ, Seo DW, Hong SB, Hong SC. Supratentorial cavernous angiomas presenting with seizures: surgical outcomes in 60 consecutive patients. Seizure. 2009;18(1):14-20.
61. Ferroli P, Casazza M, Marras C, Mendola C, Franzini A, Broggi G. Cerebral cavernomas and seizures: a retrospective study on 163 patients who underwent pure lesionectomy. Neurol Sci. 2006;26(6):390-4.
62. Yaşargil MG. Microneurosurgery, IVB: CNS Tumors: Surgical anatomy, neuropathology, neuroradiology, neurophysiology, clinical considerations, operability, treatment options. New York: Georg Thieme Verlag; 1996.

63. Chang EF, Gabriel RA, Potts MB, Garcia PA, Barbaro NM, Lawton MT. Seizure characteristics and control after microsurgical resection of supratentorial cerebral cavernous malformations. Neurosurgery. 2009;65(1):31-7; discussion 37-8.
64. Van Gompel JJ, Rubio J, Cascino GD, Worrell GA, Meyer FB. Electrocorticography-guided resection of temporal cavernoma: is electrocorticography warranted and does it alter the surgical approach? J Neurosurg. 2009;110(6):1179-85.
65. Meguins LC, Rocha da Cruz Adry RA, da Silva Júnior SC, Pereira CU, de Oliveira JG, de Morais DF, et al. Microsurgical treatment of patients with refractory epilepsy and mesial temporal cavernous malformations: Clinical experience of a tertiary epilepsy center. Surg Neurol Int. 2015;16(6):169.
66. Ozer E, Yücesoy K, Kalemci O. Demonstrated rapid growth of a corpus callosum cavernous angioma within a short period of time. J Neurosurg Sci. 2005;49(4):155-8; discussion 158.
67. Pavesi G, Causin F, Feletti A. Cavernous angioma of the corpus callosum presenting with acute psychosis. Behav Neurol. 2014;2014:243286.
68. Prada F, Saladino A, Giombini S. Trigonal cavernous angioma presenting with selective ventricular exclusion. J Neurosurg Sci. 2010;54(4):153-7.
69. Jehi LE, Palmini A, Aryal U, Coras R, Paglioli E. Cerebral cavernous malformations in the setting of focal epilepsies: pathological findings, clinical characteristics, and surgical treatment principles. Acta Neuropathol. 2014;128(1):55-65.
70. Martin NA, Wilson CB, Stein BM. Venous and cavernous malformations. In: Wilson CB, Stein BM (Eds). Intracranial Arteriovenous Malformations. Baltimore: Williams & Wilkins; 1984. pp. 234-45.
71. Sommer B, Kasper BS, Coras R, Blumcke I, Hamer HM, Buchfelder M, et al. Surgical management of epilepsy due to cerebral cavernomas using neuronavigation and intraoperative MR imaging. Neurol Res. 2013;35(10):1076-83.
72. Türe U, Harput MV, Kaya AH, Baimedi P, Firat Z, Türe H, et al. The paramedian supracerebellar-transtentorial approach to the entire length of the mediobasal temporal region: an anatomical and clinical study. Laboratory investigation. J Neurosurg. 2012;116(4):773-91.
73. Kalani MY, Lei T, Martirosyan NL, Oppenlander ME, Spetzler RF, Nakaji P. Endoscope-assisted supracerebellar transtentorial approach to the posterior medial temporal lobe for resection of cavernous malformation. Neurosurg Focus. 2016;40(Video Suppl 1):2016.1.FocusVid.15465.
74. Türe U, Pamir MN. Small petrosal approach to the middle portion of the mediobasal temporal region: technical case report. Surg Neurol. 2004;61(1):60-7; discussion 67.
75. Ding D, Starke RM, Crowley RW, Liu KC. Endoport-assisted microsurgical resection of cerebral cavernous malformations. J Clin Neurosci. 2015;22(6):1025-9.
76. Lawton MT, Golfinos JG, Spetzler RF. The contralateral transcallosal approach: experience with 32 patients. Neurosurgery. 1996;39(4):729-34; discussion 734-5.
77. Jin Y, Zhao C, Zhang S, Zhang X, Qiu Y, Jiang J. Seizure outcome after surgical resection of supratentorial cavernous malformations plus hemosiderin rim in patients with short duration of epilepsy. Clin Neurol Neurosurg. 2014;119:59-63.
78. Vale FL, Vivas AC, Manwaring J, Schoenberg MR, Benbadis SR. Temporal lobe epilepsy and cavernous malformations: surgical strategies and long-term outcomes. Acta Neurochir (Wien). 2015;157(11):1887-95; discussion 1895.
79. Upchurch K, Stern JM, Salamon N, Dewar S, Engel J Jr, Vinters HV, et al. Epileptogenic temporal cavernous malformations: operative strategies and postoperative seizure outcomes. Seizure. 2010;19(2):120-8.
80. San-Juan D, Díaz-Nuñez IC, Ojeda-Baldéz M, Barajas-Juárez VA, González Hernández I, Alonso-Vanegas M, et al. Utility of electrocorticography in the surgical treatment of cavernomas presenting with pharmacoresistant epilepsy. Epileptic Disord. 2014;16(3):245-60.
81. Menzler K, Thiel P, Hermsen A, Chen X, Benes L, Miller D, et al. The role of underlying structural cause for epilepsy classification: clinical features and prognosis in mesial temporal lobe epilepsy caused by hippocampal sclerosis versus cavernoma. Epilepsia. 2011;52(4):707-11.

Index

Page numbers followed by f refer to figure.

L

M

N

O

P

Q

R

S